# Women as Healers: Voices of Vibrancy

Tami Briggs, Editor

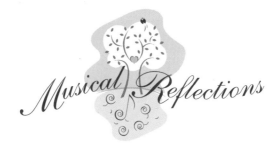

Musical Reflections Press

~Dedication~

To Aunt Carol
Who is like a sister to me and has helped immensely
on my healing journey

ISBN 0-9719822-2-8

First printing 2009

Printed in the U.S.A.

Musical Reflections Press
P.O. Box 44744
Eden Prairie, MN 55344

# Table of Contents

# Table of Contents (cont.)

# Introduction: Women as Healers
## Tami Briggs

December 13, 2008

It was an unseasonably warm, sunny day when I drove 1½ hours from my home to speak and play the harp at a "Morning of Christmas Peace" in New Richmond, Wisconsin. Every now and then, I get a feeling that "today will be very special." I had this feeling as I walked into the room where I would be speaking. It was already beautifully set up – the organizers had placed a tea cup and saucer at everyone's place setting. They had gone to estate sales, garage sales, flea markets, and rummage sales to locate 200 different cups – no two were alike, and they ranged from china cups to ceramic mugs. After I got set up, I had an opportunity to find my favorite cup – it wasn't "for the taking," but it was fun to see all of them and locate the one that appealed to me most. I made a mental note and wondered who would take that seat?

As the women started arriving, I mingled and exchanged friendly greetings. This helps me connect with my audience and, frankly, helps me to relax and relieve my nerves. When I noticed someone sitting at my favorite cup, I approached her and said, "It's so nice to meet you, and guess what?! You are sitting by the best cup!" She said, "Hi! My name is Kian and I agree. I love this cup and that's why I chose to sit here." I told her seeing Mt. Fuji and women dressed in kimonos delicately painted on the cup reminded me of living in Japan in 1987.

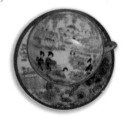

Just before I was about to speak, the organizer, Rosemary Bilgrien, came up to me and said, "There's someone who is here today who can hardly wait to meet you! Your music saved her husband's life." I was taken aback and quickly thought of a woman named Eleanor whom I had talked with on the phone back in March. She had called and wanted to order "Calm as the Night" (one of my 13 CDs). After she placed her order, she said, "I need to tell you that this CD saved my husband's life!" Well, I don't usually have people say this to me, so I asked her to tell me the story. She shared very little – her husband was a patient at a hospital in St. Paul, Minnesota, and was not expected to live. After he listened to this CD, he lived. This is really all she told me…

Rosemary asked me if we could take a break about halfway through my presentation. She had received permission from Eleanor to tell the story to the group. When Rosemary shared Eleanor's story with the group, she had more details…Eleanor's husband's doctor had told the family that they had better start preparing for his funeral, that he would not make it through the night. Eleanor and her daughters were very upset and when they went back into his room, they were sitting with him when a nurse came in and said, "I am aware of your situation. Here's a CD player and a CD called 'Calm as the Night' that might help right now."

They began playing the CD immediately, and about halfway through, Eleanor's husband squeezed her hand. When the music stopped, he opened his eyes and said, "Please turn that music back on." Needless to say, he lived through the night and Eleanor said they played the CD non-stop for two weeks!

When Rosemary finished sharing this story, I looked out at the audience with tears in my eyes; the whole group was crying. I still had an hour to speak/play; somehow, I pulled it together to finish.

After the presentation, I was standing at my exhibit table, helping those who were interested in purchasing my CDs. As the crowd was thinning, Kian appeared right in front of me and said, "I so enjoyed your stories and your music. My gift back to you – for all you gave me this morning – is this beautiful tea cup!" It was the one I had seen and admired at her place setting. I was overwhelmed with her gesture of kindness. After she purchased several CDs, she requested our picture be taken together and asked if we could meet for *tea* sometime.

After Kian and I had talked, the last two women to approach my table were Eleanor and her daughter. It was an emotional meeting.

As we were cleaning up, I mentioned to Rosemary that Kian had given me her tea cup and I told her how touched I was. She said, "Kian has an amazing story, and I hope you have a chance to meet her." I kept the tea cup on my kitchen counter for several days and e-mailed Kian asking her when we could meet. I wanted to hear her story. We met on a bitter cold Minnesota day in early February 2009. After sharing much of her story, I asked if she had told this to many people. She said she had written a few sentences, but not the complete story, in her recently published book called, *Living Your Chosen Eulogy: Live Today How You Want to be Remembered.*

For several years, I had had an idea to write a book about women as healers. I have met so many wonderful women from all over the world who are doing extraordinary work and have remarkable stories to share. As I drove home from meeting Kian, I knew I needed to share her story, as well as many others. This was a project that had to be manifested in the Year 2009! (Her story is on page 180.)

I "noodled" on the idea of this book for another six months and on July 12 – a beautiful summer Sunday morning – I went to my favorite coffee shop. I had planned to relax and enjoy the beautiful weather. Instead, I felt "directed" to hurry home and get going on the book! At 10 a.m., I began writing the invitation letter, two sample stories, and a letter explaining the details of the project for those who "accepted" the invitation. I finished at 11:30 p.m. with breaks for two meals. The words just poured out of me … it was obviously time to embark on this most special project!

The next day, I sent out more than 50 invitations with a tight timeline so the book would be complete in time for the 2009 holiday season. This meant the stories would have to be returned by August 19th – my 50th birthday! The responses from 31 women were overwhelmingly positive… what a fabulous birthday present to be gifted with all of their wonderful, heart-warming, touching stories on the milestone of 50! *Women as Healers* is part of my legacy and perhaps it is only natural for the stories to "arrive" at my half-century mark.

The contributing authors represent many facets of my life:

- Having grown up on a cattle ranch, it was destiny that I would meet Linda Rock. She is giving wonderful care and serving the same community of ranchers and their families where my beloved dad grew up.

- Having lived in Switzerland in 1982 and then five years later in Japan, it was Mary Simon Leuci who helped me recover from severe reverse culture shock twice. She and her husband also helped put the broken pieces of my heart back together when I lost a man I deeply loved and wanted to marry.

- Co-founding a cross-cultural training company with Mary Beth Lamb was an opportunity to "merge" my love for international relations with my MBA degree in marketing. For seven years, she and I had a unique opportunity to help employees doing global business to understand different cultures they were living in and working with.

- Marlou Elsen, Carien Everwijn, Vera Knezevic, Connie Fenty and I connected at a deep level at the Leading to the Edge (LTTE) conference in 2002 in Maastricht, the Netherlands. We, along with representatives from 14 other countries, envisioned a different response to Sept. 11, 2001…one of peace, not war. We continue to hold this shared vision.

- Rusty McDermott was the first to say, "Yes!" when I became interested in connecting healing music with the healthcare environment. She gave me an opportunity to be present with the lovely group of parish nurses – Jan Erlenbaugh Gaddis, Jamie Spikes, Andrea Romeiser, and Melinda Graham.

- In my earliest days of playing the harp at the hospital bedside, I "rounded" with a hospital chaplain. She told me, "You must connect with Helen Wells O'Brien." When we finally got to meet, Helen became one of my greatest teachers about spirituality.

- When I needed some context about giving care to a dear uncle with Parkinson's, Kari Berit appeared in my life…and not a moment too soon!

- The "creatives" in my life who bring sensitivity, as well as vibrancy: Janie Delaney, Connie Nelson Ahlberg, Eleanor Wiley, and Marea Whitaker Bishop.

- Holistic nurses who give extraordinary care – what an honor to watch all of them in action: Barb Schroeder, Cindy Bultena, Barb Thune Schommer, and Mary Gish.

- I greatly admire these "Passion-Brokers" who work tirelessly for their respective causes. They are making a significant contribution to the world: Judy Berry, Jackie Levin, Kay Casperson, Kian Dwyer, Ann Leach, Shashi Sharma, Jean Morrison, Mary Beth Schommer, and Cathi Lammert. They are models for all of us.

The world has much to learn from these 31 vibrant women! From Nebraska to the Netherlands, India to Iran, and Serbia to South Carolina (and many other U.S. states)…all of them are gifted healers. They, too, are leaving their legacies of teaching women to connect – to our own hearts and to each other. They are the epitome of community and a support network. It is a privilege and an honor to share their stories with you. My hope is that they touch your hearts, and that you benefit from their healing, too.

So now, I invite you to prepare a lovely cup of tea, listen to the enclosed harp CD, and allow the following stories to inspire, motivate, and encourage you along your life's path. ♥

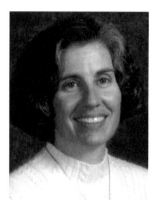

Jan Erlenbaugh Gaddis
Parish Nurse
(Faith Community Nurse)
Holy Cross Catholic Church
125 N. Oriental St.
Indianapolis, IN 46202
United States

**Phone** 317-637-2620 ext. 406

**E-mail**
jerlenbaugh@holycrossindy.org

# Jan Erlenbaugh Gaddis

Jan is a registered nurse and has worked at Riley Hospital for Children, Visiting Nurse Services, and Wishard Hospital in the Child Assessment Clinic. Since 1996, she has worked part-time at St. Francis Hospitals as the parish nurse at Holy Cross Catholic Church. She complements this nursing by working part-time at the Indiana School for the Blind and Visually Impaired as an RN in the health center.

Her educational background includes graduating from Marion County General School of Nursing (Wishard Health Services) in 1975 and completing the University of Indianapolis Parish Nurse certificate program in 1996. She also completed the certificate program at Marian College in Pastoral Leadership in 2006 and completed one unit of Clinical Pastoral Education (CPE) in 2003.

Jan's hobbies are ballroom dancing with her husband, Mike, hiking, biking, seeing movies, reading, and, surprisingly, golf(!).

# A Spiritual Awakening in Nursing

Through my life and nursing career of over 30 years, I have found myself sharing sacred moments with others, particularly at the end of life. Although I do not work as a hospice nurse, I have worked with the dying as a parish nurse for the past 13 years in a ministry of presence, healing, and wholeness. How did I come to find myself here, I ponder at times – experiencing the art and science of nursing? Then I recall those significant moments – a few in particular – in the ordinary days of work that are lasting and timeless moments remembered.

Spirituality came alive for me with Billy J, a young man of 15 years, newly diagnosed with bone cancer that had spread throughout his body. I was assigned to be his visiting home nurse. He was very much full of life until the last moments, even with all he was going through – surgery, going to school, chemo, and typical joys and struggles of boyhood approaching manhood. He did not want to be seen as disabled even though he lost his entire leg and was using crutches to catch his bus. Billy J did not like the artificial limb he was given; it slowed him down.

Billy J's last week of life was at Riley Hospital for Children in Indianapolis, Indiana. After being his nurse at home for 1½ years, I had become his "friend." I visited at his hospital bedside with his mother, and together we watched him decline physically. He inquired of everyone whether we knew what he meant by, "I'm doing my inner work preparing for my 'journey home.'" He had been confirmed in the Catholic Church by Archbishop Daniel just days before to "be made strong for the journey." At his bedside confirmation, I stood witness with him and 30 or more of his peers and friends from church. The other youth were later confirmed at the Cathedral and they remembered Billy J as a special part of the class of 1993.

A week later, I went back to the hospital to visit Billy J and his mother. His grandmother had flown to Indianapolis from New York. The nurses and doctor were at the bedside giving comfort care for him and his family. I sat on Billy J's bed holding his hand, with his mother on the other side of the bed, when he took his last breath. A tear dropped from his eye as tears rolled down my cheeks. Even in the deep sadness of loss, there was a smile on his face, and I found one on mine as his family continued to comfort each other after he was gone. When I finally left, after prayers, hugs, and goodbyes, I stepped outside to go to my car and noticed the full moon. I was in awe. I felt an intense feeling of joy and wonder, along with Billy J's presence. It was a bittersweet moment. I could not make sense of it – yet I held on to the feeling of comfort and was deeply aware that I would never do my nursing the same way again. I did not know what that meant; I just had a sense something would be different now.

I had an awakening – a sense that something bigger than me had orchestrated things in my life for the goodness of all. A few months later, during a sabbatical time away from nursing, I was aware of deep grief for so much loss in my life – not just Billy J and other patients, but family members and friends, too. I attended a workshop titled "Spirituality and Work," thinking that I needed to find new work and that it would not be in nursing. However, at this conference in upstate New York the presenter articulated, through the principles of the Creation Spirituality tradition, the "mystical experience." This is what I had experienced with Billy J the night of his death – knowing a great joy in the midst of deep sorrow. This was an affirmation that my work *is* in nursing and that I needed to find a new way of doing it.

My spirituality was awakening and developing at a deeper level. I had a lot to learn, not only about nursing and medicine, but also about spirituality and healing. I kept searching and exploring new arenas within spirituality and doing my inner work. This awakening to a deeper spirituality has continued over the years since that moment with Billy J – his final gift to me.

Along the path of spiritual exploration, of integrating faith and healing, I met other sojourners. The support I received from many people in different aspects of my life was connected, and I sensed many profound synchronistic moments. I love to learn and share at a depth that not many people find comfortable. I eventually found others who, in their own search, wanted this but could not find anyone to share with. In some way, we found each other just at the moment when we each needed to. We discovered our lives connected in response to a deeper calling from God. I had great role models and mentors, wise women and men to share my newfound questions and wonderings.

One in particular was John – a teacher, artist, mystic, seeker, a very ordinary, simple man. He had a youthful and fresh energy about him, even though he had been retired for years. He was an elder searching more and more for the meaning of life. He had seen, witnessed, and shared so much, yet he wanted to know more. He was involved in people's lives to listen and help them, but he did not know if anyone was there for him. We became partners in this spiritual journey shortly after Billy J's death – each one exploring what we needed for our own individual healing, and then to be able to help others in their journeys.

A few years later, I found myself restless again and began searching for new work. An invitation came from my church, Holy Cross: start a Parish Nurse program in partnership with an area hospital. This local facility would support a nurse who would, through an accredited course, develop health ministries and provide services for the inner-city parish community.

But first, was I qualified? They were looking at the stewardship of health and the well-being of the congregation through a holistic approach of mind, body, and spirit. The parish nurse would work toward integrating faith and health within a faith-based community. The ideal candidate would need to be a seasoned nurse and well on their way toward healing in their own spiritual journey.

The parish nurse has the role of health educator and counselor to promote healing and well-being. As a minister of health, the parish nurse is a resource/referral person. Parish nurses and health ministers provide pastoral care for the sick and dying, as well as for those who are searching for deeper meaning in their lives. The nurse walks with parishioners and offers a ministry of presence to witness God's healing work in their life. This position would involve being with people, listening to their stories, but not providing hands-on care. It would entail assisting people to tap into their own healing power within, connecting with the Divine presence.

This was a new and exciting opportunity – a new paradigm in health care. As I reflected on this unique invitation, I realized this journey perhaps started with my work with Billy J and many other patients. My friend, John, was not a patient. He was a parishioner. He, among others, walked with me in support of this new role of being the parish nurse at Holy Cross Catholic Church. This is where I find myself involved in sacred, healing work, and *being* with people in their search for wholeness. I see God working in new and surprising ways in my parishioners' lives, as well as in my own. I give a lot and receive more back. And I have become acutely aware that as I heal in my own life, this healing leads to service and giving back.

By now John was 80 years old. He had had heart trouble for many years, but since he had such a big heart, he would not give in! He was hospitalized for tests and underwent several open-heart surgeries. He never fully recovered, and developed complications. He was near death many times, and his family was asked to make the difficult decision to stop treatments for him. On the evening they gathered for their last goodbyes, I stopped by to visit and offer my support and say goodbye, as a friend and as their parish nurse. We shared prayers and stories, tears and joys. We knew John was going to a good place; he always talked about that in his many searchings. Just months before, he had self-published a simple book of his "thoughts" and reflections that he shared with his family and friends, prophetic words that would bring inspiration and comfort now in this time of letting him go.

The evening shift nurse came in to do a treatment for John. He roused just a little and opened his eyes. He slowly looked around and was surprised to see so many people at his bedside. He focused on each one with loving and caring eyes. He was not able to talk, with all the tubes attached. We knew he was smiling through those eyes and it changed the whole outlook for him and his family. There was joy amidst the bleak outlook. Later that night, his wife met with their adult children to discuss what they would do now that John had awakened. They decided to go back to the hospital room and ask him.

It was midnight. John indicated he was not ready to quit; he had too great a love of life. They decided that when John was stable, he would be moved to hospice and supported through the services there rather than be placed in a long-term care facility.

In hospice care, they were able to take him off the respirator and rid him of most all of his tubes. John thrived the short time he was there; he wanted to get better and go home "after I learn to walk," he kept saying. He had started to eat little bites of food to regain strength.

Many people found hope and inspiration through John. It was considered a miracle that he woke up. He wanted to discuss what had happened to him over the previous three months, as he had no memory of that time. He shared a great love of life with anyone who visited. His awakening reawakened in me and in others an understanding of how God's healing powers in our lives can be simple and ordinary, yet so profound.

I visited several more times with John and his wife, who was courageously holding it all together through times of family turmoil. It was amazing to witness this transformation with John and his family. Because I was not part of John's family it was important for me to step back at times and allow them to do their work. As I reflected on my inner healing, I could be present and witness God's love as a friend and not be enmeshed in the family dynamics.

Although the outcome would be the same, they had time to share a month or so more of life with visits, prayers, hugs, meals, and joking with each other. With this family, laughter was a healing balm. The last time I visited John, he was sitting up in bed ready for lunch; he ate a few bites. He offered some to me, but I declined (*good* nurses do not eat off patient trays!). Later, I realized that perhaps it was the last meal we would share. Had I missed an opportunity to break bread together? I reminisced of the many lunches we had at Wendy's when we exchanged ideas of spirituality through our 15-year friendship. We talked a little after he finished his lunch; he was becoming more reflective. He voiced that he wanted to make it back to Holy Cross, his parish and childhood church home. I watched as he processed thoughts that he might not get there "just one more time." John grew quieter and tears filled his eyes as he worked out with his God whatever was to be. I sat with him in silence…no words were needed. In this tender, intimate moment, I witnessed something bigger than each of us could understand in the mystery of letting go.

We readied Holy Cross, the church where John had been baptized, to receive him back to finish the journey he had started as an infant. Life had come full circle. At his funeral, within the communion of saints, he was whole and fully among us.

After John's death, I reflected back to the night that Billy J died and all that had transpired since then. I often wonder how I am blessed to witness these moments shared in deep intimacy. Are they connected? Are they all part of one thread in the tapestry of life? How is it that our egos and all pre-conceived notions must die so that we become even more alive? Fifteen years after Billy J's death I found myself in that moment as if nothing had happened in-between; yet everything had happened, just the way it needed to.

As a minister of health, I stand in awe of the fragile and powerful things that happen in each of our lives. We live our everyday, ordinary lives, yet there are profound things we are asked to respond to. We experience extraordinary, unplanned events that are orchestrated by someone bigger than any of us. As we show up and are present to what *is*, we see the sacred in everything. May it be so. ♥

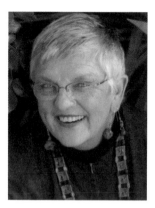

Eleanor Wiley
*Contemporary Prayer Beads*
1402 Santa Clara Ave.
Alameda, CA 94501
United States

**Phone** 510-865-1349

**E-mail** prayerbdzs@aol.com

www.prayerbdzs.com

# Eleanor Wiley

Eleanor is an artist and author, a beloved mother and grandmother. Her work celebrates the universal use of beads in prayer and the practice of being present in each moment. The Sacred Wheel of Peace®, designed by Eleanor in 1999, is her trademark. The wheel is widely accepted as "A Place to Begin," to be at peace with one another.

Eleanor has been creating contemporary prayer beads since 1994 and has presented workshops at the Parliament of World Religions in Cape Town, South Africa; Barcelona, Spain; the Balkan Youth Reconciliation Series in Plovdiv, Bulgaria; Budapest, Hungary; and Timosura, Romania. Eleanor has created personal prayer beads for His Holiness the Dalai Lama; Fr. L Freeman, OSB, founder of the World Community for Christian Meditation; Ram Das; Oprah; Rachel Naomi Remen, MD; Larry Dossey, MD, and many others.

Her books include *A String and a Prayer: Creating and Using Contemporary Beads, Beading for the Soul, There Are No Mistakes: Becoming Comfortable with Life As It Is, Not As It Should Be*, and *Changing Bead By Bead – A Present Moment Practice*.

# The Sacred Wheel of Peace®…
## A Place to Begin

Fifteen years ago, I was a speech pathologist working in long-term care when a friend asked me to help her make some necklaces. That is when I first discovered beads; today, I am known as the "Bead Lady." I create contemporary prayer beads that honor all faith traditions and cultures, and I lecture and teach around the world.

My trademark is the Sacred Wheel of Peace®…A Place to Begin; it is the foundation of my work. I designed it in 1999 as an amulet that reminds us that we must all work together if we want to move forward. The circular mandala design is intentional – the outer edge of the wheel is a representation of the rituals we practice, separated from each other. The spokes represent our spiritual path and lead to the hub in the center which allows us to be together. The

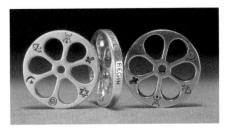

*Sacred Wheel of Peace®*

symbols were chosen as an archetypal representation of all spiritual paths.

One of my passions is to use the Sacred Wheel of Peace® and the beads to contribute to world peace. I have had the privilege of working on several peace projects – with young people in the Balkans, with prisoners in Nevada, inter-faith groups across the U.S., and many others. From the earliest days of my peace work, I had a dream of helping bring the women of Israel and Palestine towards peace. I set my intent to "make this happen" and waited for the right opportunity to present itself.

In 1999, I gave a workshop in Texas with 50 women in attendance. Because the group was large, I didn't get to know them personally. One of the women attending was Nitsan. She is the executive director of Beyond Words, a non-profit organization in Israel that works with Arab and Jewish women to promote empowerment and to help heal emotional wounds and traumas, as well as reduce prejudice that undermines the peace-building process. Two years after the workshop, Nitsan called me and asked if she could get Sacred Wheels for a group of women coming to the United States for training. I offered to do a workshop for these women, donating my teaching fee and the beads; they would pay for the Wheels and my travel expenses. We were both delighted!

Unfortunately, the person underwriting this special training in the United States lost everything in the Bernie Madoff scandal. Consequently, funding was lost and Nitsan had to say, "We cannot pay for anything. If you are able to pay your own expenses, we would love to have you come." I had to scramble and, luckily, found a couple of family members and friends to help me. I spent a wonderful day in the California sunshine with 20 women – Israelis, Palestinians, Jews, Muslims and Christians – making peace beads. They took the Wheel home to Israel…A Place to Begin.

While we were working in California, the bombing of Gaza started. One of the group members who remained at home in Gaza was killed and her family was injured. This was incredibly painful for everyone present and was a poignant reminder of the necessity of our healing work.

When Nitsan returned to Israel, she went to Gaza to visit the family. She wrote:

"I took out my Wheels of Peace® and some beads. With the help of Taha, my friend's brother, we made two necklaces – one for her daughter

Shada and one for her sister Anael. It felt so precious to be creating Wheels of Peace® necklaces with them."

I was not in Israel, but beads and the Wheel of Peace® carry my prayers. I now serve on the steering committee for Beyond Words in the United States. The Wheel® is not only in Israel, but it will be going to the Occupied Territories to be part of a workshop later in 2009. Perhaps I will travel there in 2010. This year I will have the opportunity to be in Melbourne, Australia, teaching at the Parliament of the World's Religions. At this gathering, people from many traditions will come together to make prayer beads that honor all traditions.

When I discovered beads, I had no idea how my life would change or where that path would take me. You never know where you are going to go when you start down an unknown path, but I have learned to take one step at a time. ♥

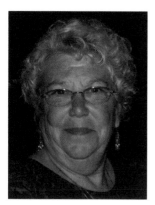

Judy Berry
CEO, *Lakeview Ranch Inc.*
69531 213th St.
Darwin, MN 55324
United States

**Phone** 1-800-546-5175

**E-mail**
lakeviewranch@yahoo.com

www.lakeviewranch.com
www.dementiacarefoundation.org

# Judy Berry

Judy is the President/CEO of *Lakeview Ranch Inc.*, Executive Director of the *Dementia Care Foundation,* and CEO of *Lakeview Ranch Healthcare LLC.* She currently owns and operates two residential homes in rural Darwin and Dassel, Minnesota, providing the Lakeview Ranch Model of Specialized Dementia Care™.

Judy has four years of post secondary education in Psychology. Judy's commitment to dementia care is reflected in her involvement at the local/regional, state, and international levels. She currently serves as a business advisory board member for Prime West Health Systems and is a regional board member for the Alzheimer's Association MN/ND branch. She is also a member of Alzheimer's Disease International (ADI) and is a consultant for the newly formed Alzheimer's Association in Nairobi, Kenya.

# Dementia Care — A Journey
# from Pain to Passion

My passion is to make a significant contribution to changing dementia care in our society and to be an advocate for all seniors with dementia.

My mother, Evelyn Holly, passed away in 1996. She spent the last seven years of her life being bounced from one nursing home or residential dementia facility to another, and in and out of hospital Geri-psych units, because of her so-called "challenging and aggressive behavior." The last year of her life, she was strapped in a chair and drugged to make her "compliant" in her environment. I spent many years of heartache and frustration struggling to find appropriate care for my mother and in the end, never found a facility to meet her needs. This link is a video of my personal struggle that fueled my passion: www.dementiacarefoundation.org/history.htm.

After my personal ordeal with my mother, I knew what needed to be done and I envisioned a dignified care model for those with dementia. However, I was told repeatedly by others in the healthcare industry that my idea was impossible because it was too expensive. It became my mission to pursue this. I could not find any financial support to try something different. So I decided to use my life savings to develop a unique model of specialized care that would focus on the unmet emotional, physical, and spiritual needs of persons with dementia. In 1999, I left my job as a Regional Sales Manager for a BBQ rib company, and at age 55 I became the founder, owner, and

CEO of Lakeview Ranch Inc. I started this project with the help of 15 seasoned health care workers.

Ten years later, we have two residential homes in rural Minnesota that people with dementia, and their families, can call "home." We focus on each resident's remaining abilities, allowing for the highest quality of life possible, while maintaining dignity and individual choice. Our current highly skilled staff of 80

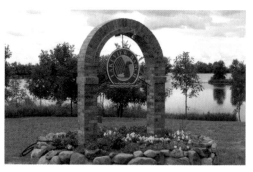

*Welcome sign to Lakeview Ranch*

provides the residents with the tender, gentle care I longed to find for my mother. My vision became a reality! Our model incorporates:

1. High staff to resident ratios (one staff member to every three residents).
2. Frequent, rigorous staff training (using specialized curricula).
3. In-house direct RN coverage for individualized, proactive disease management, and direct interdisciplinary care coordination with physicians, families, social services, etc.
4. Engaging activities such as animal therapy, music therapy, special outings, and intergenerational activities.
5. Compassionate palliative and end-of-life care for both the residents and their families.

Recent research using the Lakeview Ranch model has proven a 93.3% reduction in behavior-related hospitalizations and 36.1% reduction in the use of psychotropic medications. We are encouraged by the outcome from this research; it shows that our model works with the population of dementia and Alzheimer's patients.

From the beginning, I chose to serve all persons with dementia regardless of their financial ability. Once I had depleted my life savings, I had to find another way to provide this level of appropriate care; I refused to cut staff levels or the specialized training because both of these were very effective for our residents and families. It is a continual challenge to change the appropriation of healthcare funding from a reactive model of dementia care to proactive models that specialize in appropriate, high quality care for dementia patients. Since the U.S. government only pays two-thirds of what it costs to provide this level of care, I decided to raise money via The Dementia Care Foundation, a non-profit organization to provide scholarship funding.

Dementia is a global issue. Families all over the world are experiencing the same frustrations and pain when it comes to accessing appropriate services and support when caring for a loved one with dementia. As we reduce the illness burden to our loved ones, we help them experience a happier, safer, more secure end-of-life journey, while also significantly reducing the overall economic burden of this devastating disease.

On a recent trip to Nairobi I had the opportunity to meet with Dr. David Ndetei, Director of the Africa Mental Health Foundation, and learned of his passion to provide support and education to families there who are touched by dementia and Alzheimer's. We found we could partner in the area of access to information about the disease and support to disseminate the information in a way that is culturally acceptable.

I find it heart-warming to recognize what we can accomplish when people with vision and passion work together. We can change the face of dementia care in America and around the world — this is my on-going mission and passion. ♥

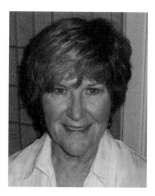

Connie Fenty
29 Golf Club Dr.
Langhorne, PA 19047
United States

**Phone** 215-906-2275

**E-mail** ConnieFenty@gmail.com

www.yournatureconnection.com

# Connie Fenty

Connie has shared her love of the Earth and passion for peace with thousands of children and adults alike in her various professional roles. As a teacher, Connie created a peace curriculum called "Winning Solutions" to educate young children about respecting others, managing anger, and solving conflicts using the "Peace Maze," a labyrinth she painted on the school playground.

As founder of *Your Nature Connection Seminars*, Connie designs and facilitates workshops on the healing relationship between people, nature, and spirit. She is a presenter both nationally and internationally.

Connie is a member of the International Labyrinth Society and serves on its Board of Directors. Her originally designed "Common Ground Labyrinth" was selected by the Society to be included in its entry to the World Trade Center Memorial Competition.

Connie also teaches a gentle yoga practice that includes reflections on inner, outer, and world peace. Her tours of England's stone circles and historical sacred sites were praised as being "life-changing."

# Heart-Shaped Healing

The lives of Nancy and Arlene, though brief and troubled, became an inspiration for Carol to create a Healing Garden at the Bucks County Women's Recovery center. The center is a residential facility providing services and housing for women who are committed to turning away from drugs and alcohol. While Nancy and Arlene had been residents there, Carol had grown fond of them and was saddened to hear that each had succumbed to their disease of addiction after leaving the safe shelter of the center.

Carol felt it was important to have a caring tribute present for the two women who struggled unsuccessfully to stay on the path of sobriety. She remembered that each had had a passion. One was an avid gardener and the other one had a walking practice. Carol decided that a labyrinth would be a perfect memorial to them, as well as providing a meditative and healing pathway for the center's current residents.

The manifestation of the Heart-Shaped Healing Labyrinth at the center is one example of the magic of synchronicity and connectivity that we healers have become accustomed to. It begins with the first chapter of my own healing journey exactly ten years ago.

While wading in the pristine tree-lined Tohickon Creek back then, I reflected with angst on the emotionally charged turbulence within my marriage. Oh, how I yearned for steady ground to stand upon. As if on cue, a still pond appeared on the land beyond the shoreline of the creek.

I stepped out of the swirling rapids of the creek to inspect the peaceful pond waters. On the ground nearby, I spotted a stone-lined circular trail that triggered a remembrance. The intriguing pattern reminded me of a labyrinth picture that I had once seen years ago. I stepped onto its winding pathway and began a restorative meditative walk. I felt instant relief as I sensed the support of solid ground beneath me.

During the years that followed my "discovery," the labyrinth has become a constant companion and healing modality for me and countless others who step upon its sacred path. An ancient symbol, mysterious in its history, the labyrinth connects us to ancestors who have made the same journey. Acting as a container of expanded space and time, the labyrinth allows us to slow down, move in a circular flow, and be led to its center as well as to our own.

My first public offering as a self-made labyrinth designer, installer, and workshop facilitator took place in my own backyard. I had laid out twinkling clear Christmas lights on my lawn in the classic seven-circuit labyrinth pattern and invited friends to enjoy a "Full Moon Labyrinth Walk." The monthly moon walk became a time when we gathered for sharing about our lives and to tell the stories of what had happened to us while in the labyrinth.

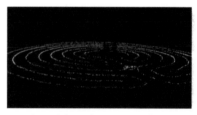

*Classic labyrinth pattern made with twinkling lights*

It was at one of these early gatherings that I met Carol. We lost touch when I eventually divorced and sold my house. It was with sadness that I removed the lights from the lawn and closed that chapter of my labyrinth journey. Joyously, those same lights reappeared later on a very large labyrinth created for a nearby recreational farm where hundreds of local people walked its illuminated paths.

One of my favorite ways of sharing the labyrinth then was to pack up my portable rope version and attend conferences where I would lay out the pathways and facilitate a workshop for participants. At an international conference in the Netherlands, I met Tami Briggs, a therapeutic harpist from Minnesota. We recognized one another as kindred spirits and have remained long-distance friends since then.

On a tour bus in England a few years after our initial meeting, Tami and I collaborated on a heart-shaped labyrinth pattern that she intended to use on a CD of original harp music. That same pattern now rests on the lawn of the Women's Recovery Center.

Recently, a friend named Carolyn attended one of my resurrected Full Moon Walks now being held at a local spiritual goods store and gathering space for holistic workshops. At the time, I was unaware that she was also a friend of Carol, the director of the Women's Recovery Center. When Carolyn visited the Center, she was still processing her "moon walk" and shared with Carol about the experience. Carol was delighted to hear that she could finally contact me regarding the installation of her meditation garden labyrinth.

At our first meeting, Carol and the residents decided the pattern best suited to their purposes was that of the Heart-Shaped Healing Labyrinth. On a Saturday morning a few weeks later, we had a busy workday and completed a template of the labyrinth by attaching rope to the ground with roofing nails, a sort of acupuncture for the earth. Pride was evident in the faces of the residents whose hands-on involvement had cooperatively created the special sacred space.

Collective awe was present as we ceremonially opened the labyrinth and were led in by the senior resident carrying a candle. The newest resident entered last carrying a Twelve Step book and reading from it when all had gathered in the center. Tears flowed when one of us noted that we totaled 12 women standing there in the middle of the concentric hearts of the labyrinth.

Those courageous women, each committed to healing her life,

continued to work together during the next weeks to replace the rope lines with bricks and add plants, hand-made tiles, and sitting benches to their garden. They finished just in time for a public dedication.

On a cool and breezy summer evening, over 40 people attended the event and walked the labyrinth. It was a tribute to its creators: all of us mentioned in this story. When it was time to go, I was about to blow out the candle at the entrance in its crystal holder when I noticed there were two flames inside glowing side by side.

As we viewed what appeared to be a miracle, I heard Carol state from a deep well of knowing, "Nancy and Arlene are at peace."

Key learning: "Although our life's journey may sometimes wind us away from our center, if we trust our path, it will eventually take us there: to our essential self." ♥

# Linda Rock

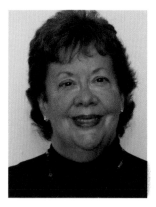

Linda L. Rock
Executive Director
*Prairie Haven Hospice*
2 West 42nd Street, Suite 2300
Scottsbluff, NE 69361
United States

**Phone** 308-630-1149

**E-mail** rockl@rwmc.net

www.rwmc.net/body.cfm?id=35

Linda is the Executive Director of *Prairie Haven Hospice* in Scottsbluff, Nebraska. *Prairie Haven Hospice* is a community based, not-for-profit, comprehensive care program for individuals with terminal illnesses and their individuals' families. *Prairie Haven* serves nine counties in western Nebraska and eastern Wyoming through three offices. Under her direction, the program has grown from serving approximately 70 patients/families per year to serving more than 500 patients/families per year and has tripled its service area.

Linda's commitment to hospice is reflected in her involvement at the local/regional, state, and national levels. She is a member of the Nebraska Hospice and Palliative Care Partnership and currently serves on the Operations Committee. She is a current member of the Regional West Medical Center Bioethics Committee and serves as a CASA (Court Appointed Special Advocate) volunteer for Scottsbluff County.

On a national level, Linda currently serves on the National Hospice and Palliative Care Organization (NHPCO) board of directors as the Central Plains geographic area representative. She chairs the Professional Education Committee, as well as serves on NHPCO's board of directors Executive Committee and is secretary of the board.

Linda has a BA degree in Sociology and Psychology from Central Michigan University. She is married with three adult children.

# Abide with Me

Margaret and I sat together in her living room looking out her picture window at acres of wheat and a herd of cattle grazing in the pasture. In a voice weakened by her battle with respiratory disease, she shared her family's history and their life on the ranch. She raged at her debilitated and ravaged body, questioned her value in life, and pondered when her death would come. She intermittently cried and laughed. I held her hand, listened, simply *abiding* with her, offering no clichés or soothing words. As I was preparing to leave, Margaret offered me a hug and said, "Thank you for remembering that I am a person, not a disease, not a patient, but a person."

I became involved in hospice care in the early 1980's, first as a volunteer and then as a board member. I believed that dying people deserved a level of care that was not available to them in home care, hospitals, or nursing home facilities. I believed that people at the end of their lives deserved care that served the person not the disease, met their physical, emotional, and spiritual needs, and also provided support to their loved ones. Too many times in my work with the chronically ill, I saw people dying alone and in pain, and their loved ones left to grieve without support. I witnessed health care providers struggling with how to care for dying patients, and saw them grieving, also. I knew there had to be a better way. That better way was and is hospice.

In my current position as Executive Director of Prairie Haven Hospice, a program serving over 9,000 square miles in rural western Nebraska and eastern Wyoming, I have the privilege of *abiding* with and learning from countless individuals who are facing the end of their lives. These individuals and their families embody grace, dignity, courage, and hope. They teach me how to live each day with joy and optimism. While all the expertise we offer in the way of pain and symptom management contributes to patients' and families' quality of life, I have discovered that nothing we do in hospice means more than honoring those we serve, respecting their uniqueness, and *abiding* with them as they complete their life's journey.

Sharon and I had a long talk at her kitchen table one snowy morning just before dawn. The hospice nurse was with Sharon's husband tending to his pain. Sharon shared that she was overwhelmed by the work she now had to do to keep the farm going and was terrified about what the future would hold. She was reluctant to share these feelings because she thought it made her seem weak and uncaring. She did not want Pete to know how frightened she was. I simply let Sharon talk, offering only an occasional encouraging word to let her know I was *abiding* with her. As she talked she became less anxious and began to formulate a plan about how she would manage the farm. Over the next few weeks, she shared that plan with Pete and asked for his input and guidance. Together they grieved but also, as in the years past, they partnered to solve their challenges. Pete voiced gratitude that he could still be of value and help to Sharon; she felt much less alone and not as frightened.

In rural communities, we are often caring for our friends and neighbors. We are called upon to offer the very best of ourselves as people face the end of their lives. We are providing that care across vast distances and over terrains that are beautiful, yet challenging. We have the privilege of serving varied cultures including people of Hispanic, Native American, and Asian heritage. Each patient and family is unique and our care is provided based on that uniqueness. As the pioneers who settled this land were, we must be creative and resourceful as we deliver our care and services.

In my daily work, I am constantly reminded that life is precious and a life is not measured in how many days one lives, but in the manner in which those days are lived. I strive every day to live all the days of my life. ♥

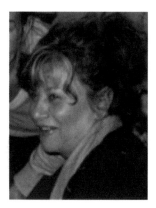

Janie Delaney
*Janie Delaney, Inc.*
1315 Woodhill Ave.
Wayzata, MN 55391
United States

**Phone** 952-473-4666

**E-mail** janie@janieinc.com

# Janie Delaney

Janie is first and foremost a mother and grandmother. She is also president and owner of *Janie Delaney, Inc.*, a successful graphic design company located in Wayzata, Minnesota. Janie's background is varied, and includes massage therapy, Reiki, gardening, and golf course greens keeper. She is intrigued and interested in alternative thoughts, ideas, and therapies, and loves working with elders. Janie loves junk, garage sales, and recycling. She is searching for her next niche.

# Every Ending has a Beginning

I'm in the hospital's water birthing room in St. Paul, Minnesota on the evening of September 23, 2008. Dim light. Nearly silent. A green iridescent light glows from the iPod playing harp music. I think to myself, "Am I supposed to be here?" I am waiting and wondering what my role is here.

Annie, my only child, and her husband, Ted, had called from Africa months earlier to tell me they were expecting a baby, and now the day had arrived. Months of Hypno-Birthing® classes, hours of meditation and breathing, wouldn't prepare Annie or Ted or me for how the birth of Delaney could change lives and remind so many of new beginnings and, yes, endings, too.

As it is with most families, babies come home and parents are raw from sleepless nights. Grandparents cook and clean and reassure and keep a low profile; again I asked, "What was my role?"

As time went by, I thought I was understanding what it took to be a grandma…just "be there." Have a hand ready, cook, bake something. But most of all, relieve the new parents for an hour or two until their much-needed time away turns into an early return because they can't wait to get back…in our case to see Dell (Delly, as we called her) because they missed her!

While the wonderment of Delly's arrival was still fresh, my mom, Ann

– Delly's great-grandma – was slowly relinquishing her role. Mom still looked like a grandma, but had long forgotten she was one. The ravaging effects of Alzheimer's disease had taken over and Delly would never have the chance to really know her. However, in the months after her birth, Delly did have time to be with her great-grandma in her recliner. There were "moments" when mom made the connection and I know it was Dell who ignited that momentary spark. They "connected."

Several months later, Dell, Annie, and I spent the last two days of Ann's life on a blow-up bed next to her hospital bed. Dell napped peacefully next to Ann during her last hours. Four generations. Ann and Dell like two bookends, holding up the generations in between…Annie and me.

Did mom know we were all there? Will Delly know what a gift it was to witness all of us together and what strength it brought us?

I realized shortly after mom's death that I had forgotten to ask her questions about being a grandma, because it just hadn't occurred to me that I should ask, or that I would be a grandma any time soon. Now I know the conversation never needed to take place. I realize that being a grandma isn't a lesson read or taught or discussed. It is woven between generations like a golden braid…strand over strand. It evolves. It's innate. The stories are our own…grandma and grandchild. Just as Annie will have stories about time spent with her grandchild…so will Delly.

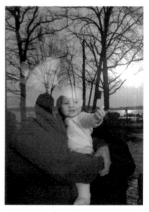

*Annie and Delly the day after mom's funeral.*
*Is that mom's light in the sky?*

I relished the stories I had come to know of big Annie, my mom, and little Annie, my daughter, and their time together…simple, yet authentic and lasting.

Mom would let Annie "style" her "just-done" hair into some ridiculous "do." She'd let her do a makeover with so much blue eye shadow, blush, and red lipstick that mom looked like a clown. Mom didn't wash it off because, in little Annie's eyes, she was beautiful. Mom taught Annie to make "wedge" salads before they became a fine restaurant menu item. The two of them played board games and had popcorn and Diet Coke on nights while they watched "their" favorite show, *Star Search*. The two of them shared *Special K* bars, lakeside overnights and late night "sleep-overs," and sayings like "a-ring-a-ding-ding and a bottle of rum," plus a few swear words! And they shared so much more. My mom, Annie's Grandma, was the epitome of what a G-woman should be. It was about love and loving it. Annie remembers big eyeglasses from the '80's and mom's "black hole of Calcutta" on the top of grandma's hair. Anyone who has one will know what it means.

Annie and mom had their own special brand of love, and I know I will have that with Delly because we are another beginning. I am now the oldest on this maternal side of my granddaughter's life…this has been bestowed upon me by my mom's passing. I will get a new hairdo, a makeover, eat *Special K* bars, and Delly and I will have our own special times just like my mom and Annie had. We'll maybe swear a little and sing "Delly-Wellie Doodle All Day" when we are doing something naughty and laughing all the way!

So the stories continue. A beginning…an ending…a beginning…an ending…

Just like with royalty…the title is handed down, only this time it's the title of "grandma." Thank you, mom, for handing me the title of "grandma." Thank you, Annie, for being a daughter, and Delly, for being a granddaughter. I love you and I will do my best to leave you memories.

Love. Love. Love.
Grand "ma" Janie ♥

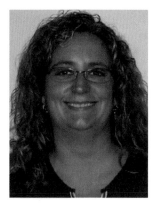

Andrea Romeiser
50 Palomino
Cape Fair, MO 65624
United States

**Phone** 417-846-3312

**E-mail** anyaro73@yahoo.com

# Andrea Romeiser

Andrea is a registered nurse who works as a charge nurse on a surgical floor where many women have had mastectomies. Andrea and her family have moved from flat rural western Kansas to the hilly country of the Missouri Ozarks. Family, friends, and the Relay for Life take her and her family back to Kansas to continue to Celebrate Life. Andrea plans to continue her involvement with the Relay in Kansas and in Missouri, and also to initiate her Parish Nurse Ministry with her new church family.

# Cooking up a Cure for Breast Cancer

In the spring of 2003, my health took an unexpected turn when I was diagnosed with breast cancer. This story is not only about my continual healing process from the disease, but also what the journey taught me. Any cook will tell you that in order to succeed in the restaurant business you need a quality support staff. My group of family members, best friends, my parish nursing group, Vegas buddies, high school friends, and college friends was called the Spice of Life Team. Without them, I would not be the individual I am today.

Even before being diagnosed with cancer, healing others had always been an interest of mine. I am the oldest of four; my youngest brother, Brian is physically and mentally challenged, and he has been my inspiration for becoming a nurse and doing healing work. After completing my nursing degree at Fort Hays State University in Hays, Kansas, I began my career at Hays Medical Center. This is a special hospital campus located on the prairie with the goal of being "the best tertiary care facility in the United States."

Even though I was happily married and had two beautiful daughters (yes, I'm a bit prejudiced!), I began yearning for an occupational change. Almost on cue, I discovered parish nursing, which would allow me to work with the community and help those less fortunate. I wrote a grant so that I could go through the training program and begin incorporating this practice into my home church. In the spring of 2003, I also became a hospice volunteer. In the late spring or early summer, I noticed a piece of skin starting to flake and peel on my right breast. I mentioned this to my husband and said jokingly, "It might be breast cancer." His reply, "Don't be silly." We didn't say another word about it.

When I attended the Parish Nurse training program in the summer of 2003, one classmate, Joan, from Wichita, had just finished her last chemotherapy treatment for breast cancer a day prior to class. Our class of Joan, 10 others, and me bonded closely through our training experience and we received much healing, both emotionally and spiritually.

In August, I decided to get an annual physical examination. I mentioned the spot on my nipple to my doctor. I was told it was probably a callous from breast feeding. I kept telling myself and really believed that it was no big deal. In late September, I noticed it again and decided to see a breast specialist. My appointment was set for a Thursday. After the doctor examined me, she said she would have to do a biopsy and said it could possibly be a very rare type of cancer; I was reassured the chances of that were very slim. She continued that she couldn't do the biopsy that day because she didn't have the correct numbing medication in the office to do the biopsy. I was frustrated because I knew from my medical background that all she had to do was get it from the pharmacy by making a simple phone call. No – I would have to return the next day…a Friday.

As I was walking home, my neighbor, Kathy, was outside working in her garden. We visited for awhile and I warmly asked her to put me on her prayer list for the night, as I was having a simple procedure the next day. Despite my initial hesitation, she went with me to the doctor for moral support. The process of the biopsy was horrible, and I often thank Kathy for taking me because I wouldn't have been able to drive home. My husband wasn't able to pick me up because he was out of town.

A very long weekend passed. On Monday, when I finally was able to speak with the doctor, she told me the biopsy results indicated I had the very rare type of cancer we had previously discussed. The spicy cancer ingredient had made its way into my recipe. My official diagnosis was ductal carcinoma in-situ with Paget's disease; a type of breast cancer that touches only 1-2% women.

I had always felt I was special but I certainly didn't need any rare disease to prove it! Why was this happening? I was only 30 years old, and in the best shape of my life. To add to that, I had nursed both of my babies for over a year. Breast feeding is supposed to decrease the chances of breast cancer. My approach was that I just needed to share the news so prayers could start my healing process. I immediately called my husband at his job – he came home. I called my mom at work – she prayed. I started making phone calls to all my friends. Each of their responses was different. When breaking the news to my friends on the phone, I rarely cried. Lana, one of my college friends, started screaming into the phone, "This is not fair! How can you remain so calm?" I had cancer and I was going to beat it.

The weekend after my diagnosis, I attended a church service where the Parish Nursing Health Ministry was initiated. It was a healing service where members from four small Methodist Churches met for a countywide gathering. Here, my diagnosis was announced to friends, acquaintances, and members of the four congregations. I stood at the altar, received the sign of the cross on my forehead, listened to special prayers, and hugged in a long embrace with my minister, Kathy. (She is one of my closest friends and the neighbor and who drove me home from the biopsy.) With tears streaming down my cheeks, I gave my body, mind, and spirit to God, and felt an overwhelming sense of peace.

At my first doctor's appointment, we decided to remove part of the milk ducts in the right breast and then proceed with radiation. By the time the scheduled surgery date came, I was so stressed they had to give me extra medication to bring down my blood pressure; then they had a hard time waking me up. After the surgery, I received good news – the cancer had not spread into my lymph system – neither to my lymph nodes nor to the rest of my body.

However, when I went for my first follow-up after surgery, I was informed the "margins" weren't clear. (This meant a few cancer cells could possibly still be in my body.) I went back to surgery in a few days and again, the margins weren't clear. At this point, my doctor suggested I go from Hays to Wichita for a mastectomy and reconstruction to be done at the same time. Reconstruction of the breast was not available in Hays and if I went to a larger facility, both the mastectomy and reconstruction could be completed at the same time. I didn't really care about reconstruction; I just wanted all of the cancer *out* of my body. The day before Thanksgiving we went to Wichita to see a breast specialist and the plastic surgeon. They posed a lot of questions: Should I remove one breast or both? Should I have implants or use my own tissue? We had these and a lot of additional decisions to make.

There is a lot of cancer in my family history. My maternal grandmother had breast cancer in her later years, as did five of her sisters. My dad's only sister had died of breast cancer just a couple of years earlier. With that bleak family medical history in mind, I decided to have both of my breasts removed. On December 12, 2003, I had bilateral mastectomies with the insertion of tissue expanders (half empty saline implants). I was in the hospital for four days. In order to deal with the daily pain, I needed two pain pills every three to four hours. But the cancer was all removed from my body, so nothing could put a damper on my spirit.

In spite of my optimism, I didn't heal well. I had two drains that continuously drained and they ended up staying in for 54 days. Typically, the drains are used for a week or two at most, but my body kept producing enough fluid so they couldn't be removed. Then I got an infection on the left side (the side that didn't have cancer). After being very ill, I was finally hospitalized and had daily IV antibiotics. The treatment and antibiotics didn't work so it was decided that the tissue expander had to be removed. The good news was I saw an oncologist and he told me the treatment I had chosen was a good choice with the type of cancer I had. He said, "God has been watching over you. If you hadn't found the piece of skin flaking off, you could have been dead in two to five years."

Three months later, the expander was put back in. Six weeks after this surgery, my skin started to blister and my medical team decided to remove the expander once again. I had surgery to remove the expander, wash the cavity, and then put the expander back in. Eleven days later, it had to be removed…yet again.

This was a crazy time; on top of everything else, my Dad had a heart attack. So, he and I were both in the same large hospital on opposite ends of the facility. Ironically enough, that wasn't the first time my Dad and I had been sick together. While I was in college, he had a stroke and I had my tonsils removed at age 22. We are quite a pair!

It was hard to have only one tissue expander in when the other side had been stretched twice so the skin was just hanging. I had a very hard time with the visual side of breast cancer. Once when I was traveling, I used socks to fill the left side of my bra because I had forgotten the insert. It was a good laugh! After that I had two more surgeries to complete the process. I was FINALLY "fixed."

What a journey it has been! In total, I had 10 surgeries in 2½ years. During that time, I also experienced the loss of all my grandparents, my father's heart attack and two strokes, and marriage counseling. Best of all, since my diagnosis, I have celebrated each daughter's birthday six more times.

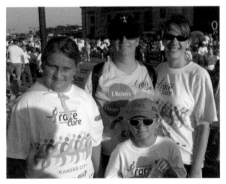

*My two daughters, Bailey and Aspen, with a friend. (I am wearing the black cap.)*

I was cured of cancer when all of it was finally removed, but I continue to heal. I have lost several friends to cancer and have more friends with a new diagnosis of cancer. My friend Lana (the one who screamed on the phone) has beat thyroid cancer, and my second mom, Woodi, has also beaten a rare type of stomach cancer.

One in three people will be affected by some type of cancer. For this reason, I have been involved with Relay for Life (www.cancer.org). The Relay for Life celebrates those who have won the fight, remembers those who have lost the fight, and energizes us all to continue to fight back for our children's future. The goal is that someday we will no longer have the word "cancer" in our vocabulary!

I helped initiate a Relay in our small county in rural Kansas (Rush County, population 3,600). We hold the 12-hour event from 7 p.m. to 7 a.m. (this timing symbolizes the long night of the cancer journey). Teams "hold vigil" around-the-clock and around the track with 3,500 luminaries lighting the path in honor and in memory of those who have fought the fight against cancer. In 2008, Rush County was #10 in the United States in money raised per capita. In June, 2009, we raised $68,852.39; this was $15,648.56 more than in 2008! This is an example of the wonderful support and great love I have felt from this community. While small in population, Rush County is mighty in the fight against cancer!

My spice of cancer was sweetened with the care of God who could not protect me from cancer itself, but could protect my life. I continue to believe He was there in the beginning and continues to help mix up my life recipe, which recently has been delectably pleasing. I pray that I may continue to enjoy this tasty recipe, and I also pray for my girls, who wear pink and proudly tell others their mom is a breast cancer survivor. I pray for my husband and me to continue the spiciness in our life. I celebrate life each and every day, and I invite you to do the same!

Everything that has affected your life is just another ingredient…I hope your recipe of life is spicy sweet! ♥

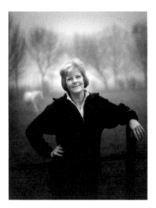

Carien Everwijn
*O'Neil Consult*
Runneboomweg 1
8131 RN Wijhe
The Netherlands

**Phone** 031-572-362818
031-655-195158

**E-mail**
carien.everwijn@wanadoo.nl

www.oneilconsult.nl

# Carien Everwijn

Carien worked in the Netherlands in human resource management at an international bank. While at the bank, she conducted workshops and trainings in Holland, England, Germany, Russia and the United States. Carien has also conducted workshops in Holland and abroad with Erik van Praag, founder of The Edge: A School for Spiritual Leadership.

After 29 years of corporate life, Carien now devotes her time to her coaching and consulting practice called *O'Neil Consult*. She lives in the country on a farm in the Netherlands doing what she loves best – helping people heal using horse therapy.

Her university studies were in Cultural Anthropology in Amsterdam.

# Healing…
# The Most Natural Thing on Earth

Why were you born? What are you doing on this earth? Peter Goldman asked these questions during a workshop that I attended in 1979. I panicked. I couldn't come up with answers. I was very angry with Peter for asking these "stupid" questions. At the time, I was 30 years old and simply wanted to be married and have children. I didn't vent my anger; I just tucked the questions away in my mind. Eventually, my life vision formed from these questions. I saw myself counseling people, somewhere on a farm, and I knew that animals and horses played an important role.

In the following years, I didn't act upon my vision, but worked in the human resources department for an international bank. My responsibilities changed over time, and eventually my office door said, "Coach-Counselor." My long-lost vision from Peter's early questions came back when Fuego, a beloved horse of mine, had to be put down. His ailments were such that there was no hope for him. His passing made me remember the powerful bond that is shared between an animal and its owner. My sorrow of losing him also led me to attend numerous workshops and trainings about becoming a counselor who uses animals for their healing abilities. During one of those trainings, I declared that I needed a therapy pony rather than a horse. "Oh," someone said, "I have one for you." And so I was offered Bella, my beautiful white healing pony.

Little did I know that I would be the first person that Bella healed! Upon first mounting her, the soles of my feet strangely came alive. It felt great. Years later at a colleague's workshop in Germany, my feet had the same experience on another horse. "Don't move. I must go get my camera!" she said while racing into the house. She saw what I felt – in that very instant everything in me was congruent, flowing, and at ease. I felt the same greatness on this horse as I did on Bella's back. Much later a friend said to me, "Don't you know that your soul enters your body through your feet?" I didn't.

Over time, Bella not only taught me more effective ways of counseling people, but also how I could aid in her job of healing others. For example, Bella often helps me, and my clients open their feet, as if to say, "Look, trust the earth, relax and surrender." Another lesson Bella taught me was how to let go of assumptions regarding "proper" counseling methods.

One of our first clients was a person who was very experienced with horses and was a life coach who helped corporate managers find fulfillment with their work. As she sat on Bella's back and walked her through our working area, Bella kept stopping. I apologized, "I'm sorry she stops all the time...I don't know why." After the session ended the client said, "I know now why she stopped. Whenever I held my breath, Bella would stand still." So we experimented with steady breathing techniques through challenging situations and I promised her that if she really let things flow inside her body, Bella would trot. And so she did! "Thanks for not telling me and letting me figure it out for myself," the client said afterwards. I couldn't have told her, but when she mentioned that she stopped breathing, I noticed that I had too. Now when I ask somebody to do energy exercises while sitting on the horse, I can follow inside my own body what's happening, which gives me different insights. In the 30 minutes that the three of us worked together, it was amazing to see how much we learned, grew, and healed!

Having Bella made it easier to leave my corporate job and work with her and clients full-time. The process of working with Bella has become easier and much faster. A number of people have been able to let go of pain simply by sitting on her for ten minutes. The two of us have helped a variety of people – from children to corporate managers – with all sorts of questions and situations. I learned to put 100% trust in Bella's reaction. I then began thinking of more exercises that would help clients let go of their knotty problems within themselves so that the healing process could begin. As this beautiful work continues to evolve and grow, more people are open to this unique form of healing.

After a few years we moved from a tiny space to the farm where we now live. Thirty years after Peter's questions, I am happy to say that I live my vision – I know why I was born and what I'm doing on this Earth! Bella's mate, Sandor, and my dog, Ollie, have taken their rightful places helping and healing those who come to the farm. Through living on the farm, I have learned to be a part of nature. The more I learn, the more I heal; the deeper I heal, the more healing I can help facilitate in others. Healing truly is the most natural thing on earth. ♥

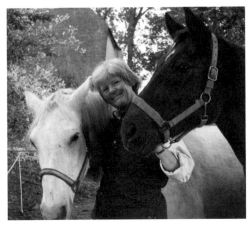

*My horses Bella and Sandor*

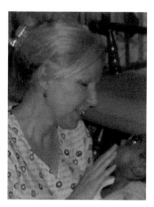

Melinda Graham
7773 South Burma Road
Smolan, KS 67456
United States

Phone 785-212-0435

E-mail
sparrowsong7@yahoo.com

# Melinda Graham

Melinda is a registered nurse and holds certification in touch/massage interventions for infants and toddlers, including those who are fragile, premature, and have special needs. After four years of study in the field of energy medicine, she is in her apprenticeship year with the Healing Touch Program and will complete certification in late 2009. She works part-time with an early intervention program providing consultation and education for the health and well-being of children with special needs and their families. Her private practice, *Sparrow Song*, will open in November 2009 and will offer a variety of gentle healing arts.

Melinda teaches and presents in a number of educational and retreat venues on touch, prayer, energy medicine, and issues regarding children with special needs. Audiences have included students, healthcare professionals, women's groups, parents, and adult learners. She has been the recipient of numerous arts and humanities grants for poetry, and has also received a healthcare grant to work with infants with GERD.

# It's All About Love

"Hey, can you help us? We've got a dad we can't get out of here. He is making us crazy with all of his questions. And I think he's making the other parents nervous because he just stares at everybody. He is pretty scary looking. His wife, Julie, is in intensive care. His baby girl is named Lilly and she was born two months premature. She is on a minimal stimulation protocol. She's stable off oxygen unless she gets touched and then she gets irritable and her oxygen saturation dives."

This plea for help came from Cathy, Lilly's nurse. She was on the 14th hour of her 10-hour shift and it showed around her eyes and in the slump of her shoulders. She drained a can of Coke and tossed it expertly into the trash can in the corner of the nurse's locker room. I had worked in this neo-natal intensive care unit (NICU) with Cathy for 18 years; I knew what it was like when it got crazy. I remembered how difficult it was to work with a parent watching, questioning everything we did.

Five years ago, I left the NICU to work with infants and toddlers with special needs. I'd recently completed training to provide touch interventions for premature and fragile infants, and massage education to their parents. As a part of the certification process, I needed to work with infants and their parents in the NICU. Tonight, I was stopping by to check on what babies I could see the next day.

As Cathy and I were about to leave the locker room, she said, "So, are you going to help us get that dad out of here? His name is Tom." Cathy must have caught the glimmer in my eye because she said, "What are you thinking? You have that *look* when you get an idea." I smiled as sweetly as I could and said, "Don't worry. Tom just needs to have a role, something he can do for his baby. He can't fix things and he has no control – that's why he won't leave and is questioning everything, right?"

"Maybe, or he's just aggressive; have you seen him?" I looked at her without expression. Cathy insisted, "What are *you* going to have him do? His baby is on minimal stimulation – he can't touch her." I raised my eyebrows and said, "Touch isn't always about moving your hands. I won't do anything that jeopardizes the baby. Trust me." Cathy covered her face with her hands; then separated her fingers and peeked out. "If that baby drops her oxygen saturation, I'm telling everybody you are a bad, bad nurse!"

As I walked into the NICU, I could see a nurse talking to a man who was sitting on a tall stool; his black leather boots planted on the lowest rung. He looked like a sentinel, a very large sentinel, positioned at the side of his baby's warmer. His black T-shirt stretched tight around his biceps and across his broad back – he as built like a rugby player. His copper-colored hair was tied with a black cord and hung midway down his back. He looked over at the warmer where his tiny daughter lay amid a jumble of patches, tubes and wires. I walked toward him and when I said his name, he turned around on the stool, and, just for an instant, I saw weariness and worry in his furrowed brow before he straightened, crossed his arms over the Harley Davidson logo on his chest, and regarded me. "What?!" His head was tipped slightly back; his grey eyes narrowed.

I introduced myself and asked about Lilly. He glanced at the warmer and back at me. "You a nurse? Why aren't you in the same color scrubs? You in charge or something?" I answered his questions. He never changed expressions. Lilly began to wiggle and scowled in her sleep; an alarm sounded above her bed. I turned toward the bed, reached up, and silenced it. I could feel him right behind me. He was well over six feet tall and was standing very close, looking over my shoulder at his daughter. "I hate that buzzer. Sometimes when it goes off, they act like it's nothing. Last night, she turned all grey and quiet when it rang and they didn't come over here very fast. How come they do that? I think that wire might scratch her arm, should it be around her arm that way? I think her nurse took a break. Where is she?" Lilly frowned. Cathy caught my eye from across the room and shook her finger at me.

As we moved away from the warmer, I told him about over stimulation and the sensitivities of monitors; I showed him how soft the wire was that he'd questioned. I told him I'd stay with Lilly until her nurse returned. He didn't say anything but walked out of the nursery, glancing back at his daughter every few steps, oblivious to the other parents and nurses moving out of his way. He was on his way to see his wife, Julie, who had moved from intensive care to the mother-baby unit.

While he was out of the nursery, I reviewed Lilly's records and then spent some time watching her reaction as I moved my hands near her body. I eventually let them rest against her skin. I moved one hand to the crown of her head and the other to her feet. She wiggled, scowled, then settled. She could handle this kind of touch.

An hour later, I was seated next to Julie's bed; her medical condition had stabilized but she was confined to bed until morning. Tom stood on the opposite side of the room, arms crossed, looking out the window. Julie was a soft spoken woman with blue-black hair and deep brown eyes. As she told me about her pregnancy and Lilly's birth, tears began to roll down her cheeks. Tom turned from the window and moved to sit next to her on the bed. He stroked her hair as she leaned against him and sobbed. He did not look up, but said angrily, "I hate this! There's not a damn thing I can do. I hate going in that place to watch my baby just lay there. Babies are supposed to cry but Lilly can't even cry – how am I supposed to take care of her?"

I let a few moments of silence pass. "Would you like to hear a prayer my Grandmother gave to me?" Julie nodded and Tom inclined his head slightly. I spoke the prayer into the room, and then wrote it, at Julie's request, on a paper towel – the only paper in the room. Then, for the next 30 minutes, I talked about the healing power of love, using touch to enhance physiological function, and comfort touch versus noxious touch. I talked about using stillness, rocking, and gentle pressure. We practiced on each other's arms and, in this way, we began to share the bond of touch among ourselves in a non-threatening way. I explained that if Lilly wasn't ready for direct touch, Tom could still provide a kind of touch through his hands by imagining the love from his heart filling his hands and cradling Lilly. At this point, Tom crossed his arms and said, "I don't know. Are you sure my hands aren't too big? Besides, it sounds kinda psycho!"

Julie took Tom's hands in hers and said, "Love is not psycho. You can do this for Lilly; you will be just like the prayer. It will be all about love."

When Tom and I went back into the nursery, we stood at the foot of the warmer. I could feel the nurses watching. He took a deep breath, uncrossed his arms, and put his big hands on either side of Lilly, about twelve inches away from her body. She was frowning, but still. Tom glanced at me. I nodded. He moved his hands slowly, his upper body stiff. Lilly shifted and he paused…then, started again. As soon as his hands touched her skin she grimaced, wiggled, and then settled. After a few seconds, I put my hands on his and gently guided him to scoop her body into the cradle of his palms. I moved my hands away. She stretched and settled back into his hands. Tom's expression softened and his shoulders began to relax. Lilly opened one eye. "She looks like Julie," he whispered. "Tell her," I said, as my hand rested briefly on his shoulder. He said, "Lilly, you look so pretty, just like your Mommy. I'm your Daddy." Tiny red headed Lilly opened her other eye and gazed intently into her Daddy's eyes. The oxygen saturation monitor climbed from 92 to 99.

When I returned to the NICU four days later, I was happy to see that Lilly was progressing well. She was considered a "grower," no longer a sick baby, and was off the open warmer, swaddled and fast asleep in a bassinette. I noticed a small frame was hanging by a pale green satin ribbon at the end of her bassinette. It contained the paper towel with my scribbled prayer...

*Dear Father, hear and bless*
*The beasts and singing birds.*
*And guard with care and tenderness,*
*Small things that have no words.*

And a single line written below

*It's all about love.* ♥

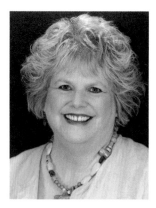

Ann Leach
2674 B Meadow Lane
Joplin, MO 64801
United States

Phone 417-624-3377

E-mail ann@life-preservers.org

www.life-preservers.org

Facebook and Twitter
Ann Leach

# Ann Leach

Ann is the founder and president of *Life Preservers: A Global Grief Support Community.* A counselor by profession, Ann has assisted hundreds of caregivers cope with a loved one's illness and death. As a freelance writer, Ann's articles have been published in regional and national magazines and business journals. She is the co-author of *Goal Sisters: Live the Life You Want with a Little Help From Your Friends* (New World Library, 2004) and is currently at work writing her next book, *Onward and Upward: Planning a Life Celebration to Remember.*

# Answering the Door
# When Death Delivered
# an Opportunity

All around me, people were crying and sending me pitying looks, and I wasn't sure why.

True, my mother had died and I was standing in the funeral home "parlor" (does anyone say "parlor" anymore?) and there were many friends who were upset, but I didn't understand the depth of their despair. It wasn't as if she had died suddenly in a car crash or on the operating table during surgery.

No, my mother died of lung cancer. She had a three-year journey that included endless treatments, multiple long distance trips to doctors' offices, regular jaunts to pick up prescriptions, and even a period of remission.

Once the cancer returned, it had its way with her, resulting in a four-day stint in the local hospice unit at our community hospital where she died. I had contacted her friends and mine the day she went into hospice and alerted them to the fact that "things don't look good," so I figured they were prepared.

Our neighbor, Helen, was one who was not.

"Honey," she called to me as she crossed the large room and closed the distance between us in only four steps. "I just feel so badly. I mean, now you truly are an orphan! And I don't know how you are going to go on like before."

Helen was a petite woman and I towered over her in stature. That night, Helen made me feel smaller than I had ever been in my life. And I was 32 years old!

I guess, though, that she was technically correct: my father had died when I was eight and I am an only child, so my mother's passing did suddenly provide me with a new title. Yet the reality of Helen's declaration was simply hot air to me.

"Helen," I said. "I am not an orphan! I have more friends that are more my family than my actual relatives ever were!" Of course, I meant no disrespect to my parents; I was really referring to the distant cousins, aunts, and uncles with whom I spoke only once or twice a year.

And who in their right mind would want to go on as before?

I knew that it was time to focus my energy on helping other caregivers cope with supporting someone who is living with cancer.

Within six months of Mom's funeral, I opened the Cancer Support Network as a center for education, support, and resources. I also pursued a Master's degree in Psychology and Counseling, working with cancer and AIDS patients, substance abusers, and others needing assistance in breaking old habits and setting their sights on something better for themselves and their lives. I provided counseling as clients coped with the loss of their old ways and the relationships that needed to be left behind in order to thrive.

My mother's death had shown me that life is indeed short and that we must truly value each moment we've been given. Why didn't everybody understand that? Why couldn't we celebrate each small step on the way to a great life?

And why couldn't we plan for an amazing life celebration when the end of that life came?

Fast forward 20 years when my focus shifted once again and I finally said "yes" to my true calling: assisting people in shifting their beliefs about death from those of fear and dread to acceptance and celebration.

Has it been an easy leap to make? Yes and no. I see now that there is nothing I would rather be doing. It is in the "doing" that I question all the usual things that attempt to stand in the way of living, and having, our dream: time, money, learning curves, marketing, and so forth. But just as I start to doubt, I meet someone who needs Life Preservers' services or offers just the right word of encouragement, and I know that this is mine to do.

Death and loss can be great teachers. I am willing to hear their lessons and guide others in appreciating them, too.

After all, we're each headed onward and upward. ♥

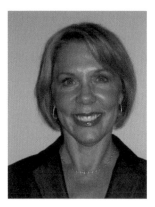

Jean Morrison
*Morrison & Associates, Inc.*
3815 Glenhurst Ave. S.
St. Louis Park, MN 55416
United States

**Phone** 952-927-9133

**E-mail**
JMhumanresources@aol.com

# Jean Morrison

Jean is President of *Morrison & Associates, Inc.*, a human resource management consulting firm. She specializes in conflict resolution, executive/individual coaching, leadership development, team building, employer/employee relations, performance and people management, and organizational change. In addition, Jean is a founding partner of *RESOLVE*, a consulting firm providing conflict management and professional training and development services.

Jean has been an instructor at the University of Minnesota for twenty years in the areas of communications, conflict management, human resource management, and performance management. Prior to founding *Morrison & Associates, Inc.*, Jean held key management and officer positions with Pillsbury, Green Giant, Michigan National Bank, St. Joseph Bank & Trust, and Norwest Bank.

Jean is a volunteer mediator for The Minneapolis Mediation Program and a mentor at the Metropolitan Economic Development Association and Bethune Elementary School.

# The Worst and Best Week of my Life

Losing my job and my health in the same week in 1986 was devastating. I was a successful, exhausted, caring, over-committed workaholic who was identified as "high-potential" by corporate executives and whose future as a human resource executive held great promise.

My workaholism had clouded my perspective and judgment and perhaps, as one practitioner suggested, may have contributed to my cancer.

After three successful surgeries, I embarked on a journey of self discovery, self forgiveness and self love. I needed to learn who I was outside of my business card title, and how to nurture the spiritual, emotional, physical, and relational aspects of myself. This was a painful and wonderful time in my life. I became a better sister, daughter, aunt, mom (to dogs), neighbor, and volunteer as a result.

As I was living more awake, engaged in life, and open to the messages and lessons life was sending me, I noticed a small ad in the newspaper for volunteer mediators for a new community mediation program. It caught my eye because mediating and resolving conflicts was something I was good at and comfortable with and had been doing throughout my career in human resources. It also seemed to be a fit because my college degrees had prepared me for working in the diplomatic arena internationally.

After a 10-week training program, a co-mediator and I were scheduled for our first mediation session – a conflict between two neighbors. The four of us met at a meeting room in a local library. The two neighbors, Bud and Roy, hadn't met before. After explaining the ground rules for mediation, we asked Bud, who submitted the complaint, to explain his side of the story. He said he had moved into the neighborhood several months before and felt very unwelcome. He was Jewish in a traditionally non-Jewish neighborhood and was certain the neighbors were anti-Semitic and didn't want him there. He waved several times to his neighbors, including Roy, his next door neighbor, and got no response.

The problem at hand was a large branch which had fallen from Roy's tree onto Bud's fence and was partially blocking his sidewalk and driveway. He waited for several weeks for Roy to clear the branch from his property but it never happened. He therefore sought help through the community mediation process. Bud said angrily to Roy, "You're disrespecting me and my property because of who I am! I have a right to live here. Who do you think you are to treat me so poorly?"

Roy sat quietly and looked down at his lap. He softly explained, "I'm sorry, I didn't notice the branch had fallen. I guess I've been pre-occupied and sort of in a fog lately. I'm taking care of my terminally ill wife, Lois, and have been burning the candle at both ends. Taking care of Lois, running errands and keeping up with the house chores has tired me out. We didn't have children and our relatives are out of town, so I'm going it alone. I want you to know that I don't know what your religious beliefs are and it makes no difference to me. I'll go home and take a look at the branch and see what it will take to have it removed right away."

Bud reached over and ripped up the document his complaint was written on and then reached out to shake Roy's hand and said, "Don't worry about it. It's okay." As Roy shook Bud's hand, he said, "Welcome to the neighborhood. It's a nice neighborhood."

When they got back to the neighborhood together, they pulled the branch off of the fence onto the grass where they sawed it up together.

My experience as a volunteer mediator began my 23-year journey as a student of conflict and conflict resolution. After repeatedly experiencing the peace and progress that can result from understanding one another, I co-founded a conflict resolution and training company called RESOLVE in 1987. I have taught a course on conflict management at the University of Minnesota for 20 years, and I consult with individuals, companies, and institutions to bring peace and understanding to the workplace for individual and organizational effectiveness.

I am grateful for the pain of the difficult week I experienced in 1986 because it helped me to discover the true essence of myself and re-set my life course. ♥

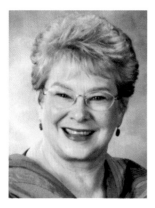

Dr. Jamie Spikes
3901 Snowy Reach
Manhattan, KS 66503-7759
United States

**Phone** 785-537-3929

**E-mail** jamiespikes@gmail.com

# Dr. Janice (Jamie) Morrison Spikes

Jamie is a registered nurse and has worked or taught as a maternal infant nurse and nurse educator in more than 10 hospitals with birth rates from 20/month to 600/month. She has practiced in areas from older adult ambulatory care services to neonatal intensive care units in four states.

In the community setting, she has been a parish nurse over 20 years and is a founding member of the Board of Management of Lutheran Parish Nurses International. She has been a long-time member of the International Alliance for Invitational Education.

Jamie is an entertaining and frequent speaker for both professional and lay groups.

Jamie and Frank have been married for 38 years. They have one son, Jonathan.

# From Paper Nursing Cap to
# Gold Tassel Mortar Board

Take an ecru wide-lined piece of Big Chief tablet paper, blunt-end scissors, make a couple folds in the paper, use a little Scotch tape, and what do you have? When you are a four year-old girl with a dream, you are a nurse wearing your very own nursing cap! I spent a full year wearing a tablet paper nursing cap until Grandma Tholen made me a *real* cotton, stiffly starched, made-to-fit nursing cap when I was five. Grandma made nurses' caps for both of Mom's sisters who were registered nurses. I wore mine proudly and regally for another two years – to me, it was a priceless tiara. And as a nurse, I had patients, too.

The most cooperative patients under my care were dolls, mostly baby dolls as I was playing with dolls long before Barbie. And besides, Barbie, Ken, and their friends would not have lowered themselves to care provided by a four-, five-, or six-year-old paper-then-cotton cap wearing nurse. Dolls welcomed bandages of various materials, tapes, and sizes and wore them for days. Dolls (and the nurse's mother) did not like mercurochrome as a primary treatment because it stained 1950's rubber doll limbs and faces; however, watercolors and crayons worked almost as well for fake lesions and wounds.

The live patients were only moderately cooperative and modestly appreciative of my care. My trusty sidekick of a cat named Jingle Bell and her numerous litters of kittens were all under my watchful healing eye. Jingle Bell and I had an understanding. First, she was *not* one of my patients. Second, as soon as her kittens were weaned, I started feeding them milk from doll bottles with large holes cut into the ends of the nipples, *and* I dressed them in doll clothes. The kittens, both female and male since I was not gender biased, wore pastel dresses with matching bonnets and bandages. They had no tolerance for booties or dressings on their paws, but they didn't seem to mind limbs being wrapped. A little gauze goes a long way on a tiny kitten arm. There was another dressing that was not tolerated and tried only once – a Band-Aid® on a kitten's leg. I could have gotten very sick from Cat Scratch Fever removing the well adhering tape. Actually, that kitten didn't want to play patient much after that incident, but I still loved being a nurse.

Along with being an outstanding nurse, I was an exceptional mother to my family of dolls. Even then I was transculturally sensitive and had both a white and a black Betsy Wetsy. The Betsy Wetsy dolls were experiential and reality-oriented in nature. If one fed them water from a bottle, in a very short time one got to change a diaper. If one forgot about the diaper or used Kleenex® instead of several thick layers of cotton, one's lap got wet. There were other things to learn from Betsy Wetsy, too. If one put something other than water in the dolls' bottle there were negative consequences. First, if one used milk, as one decided to do one day, and not all of the milk went all the way through the doll's "digestive system," the doll smelled like sour milk for days and days. Copious amounts of water were needed for a satisfactory cleansing. This was not good, so the exceptional mother did that only once.

My next idea for some white liquid resembling milk was to feed the dolls a mixture of a little flour in water. The more flour I used the more milk-like it looked. This seemed like a splendid idea! There was not much problem getting this into the dolls since the nipples on the bottles were the same ones with the big holes used for all of the kittens. However, this milk-like substance caused "constipation" for the two Betsy Wetsys since the paste went in OK, but didn't come out. Over time, the paste hardened, became "plaque" and once broken up came out as powder. All of this told me that bottle feeding the Betsy Wetsy babies was too much work on both ends, so I turned to breastfeeding. It took much less time and effort since I could "feed" both Betsy Wetsy babies at once. They seemed much more satisfied, too, and I loved being a mother.

Besides being the outstanding nurse and exceptional mother, I was also a 4-6 year old exemplary teacher. Not having had preschool or kindergarten, I knew only about Sunday School as an educational venue. In the playroom, I lined up all my dolls for class. They often looked more like patients in the waiting room of a pediatric trauma center with all of their bandages and dressings than healthy children dressed in their Sunday best for Sunday School, but they were my class. My favorite early childhood Sunday School teacher was Mrs. Fox, and I taught just like she did. The class was led in all the songs I knew, and they listened to all the memory verses I could recite. As with every good teacher at the time, I even had a flannel graph and used handmade sand paper Bible character and animal cut-outs to stick on the flannel board for the lessons. The class was very attentive to me, unlike some of those in Mrs. Fox's class. I loved being a teacher.

Using the above childhood template to lay over my adult life, the fit is hand-in-glove. My nursing career from student in the mid-1960s to professor 45 years later has been a fabulous ride. The various roles in the different settings I have had during those years have been from heart warming to heart wrenching. Since most of my clinical practice has been in maternal child, women's health, and family nursing, the opportunities for peak and valley experiences have been legion. I have been at the bedside with laboring women for hours as they brought forth their lustily crying, healthy, and ready-to-eat newborns. For some of the other mothers I have attended, their babies were born "peacefully sleeping." The joy in a delivery room is incomparable as is the grief that can be felt there. As a nurse, I have been blessed to have a therapeutic presence that helps families to heal in these life-changing moments. In retrospect, I've wondered if I've come from a line of nurse healers with a heritage for women, infants and families, as both of my grandmothers were midwives in their rural Midwestern communities in the early 1900s.

Other roles and settings of my practice have been as a staff and charge hospital nurse, camp nurse, office (obstetric and urology) nurse, school (parochial and public) nurse, and parish (faith community) nurse. Additionally, I have been a Sudden Infant Death Syndrome counselor, poison control investigator, adolescent pregnancy and birthing room researcher, pregnant and parenting teen program administrator, community and university educator, lay and professional health educator, and home visitor. My own infirmities have made me a better nurse – the latest being a breast cancer survivor. I firmly believe that I have had breast cancer so that I can educate other women about early detection and screening, help them understand various treatment options, support them in their decision, and be there for them during their treatment choices. As a uniform and cap-wearing, lab coat and suit wearing, or jeans and a sweatshirt wearing nurse, I love being a nurse.

As for being a mother, my husband Frank and I have a wonderful 28-year-old son who is an officer in the U.S. Army. His role is a medical evacuation Blackhawk helicopter pilot. His formal educational preparation for this is a BA with a major of media studies in communications and minor in psychology, a master's in curriculum and instruction, and he's considering a doctoral program in student services and higher education. Prior to the army career, he enjoyed skydiving and scuba diving. Both of his parents hardly climb higher than a step stool and not much deeper in water than a bathtub! For the record, he was breastfed; however, he did take longer to feed than Betsy Wetsy, but did demonstrate the same intake and output consequences. I love being Jonathan's mother.

Going from being an invitational Sunday School teacher with a room full of dolls to a Baby Boomer university professor with a classroom full of Generation Y or Millennial nursing students has been quite a leap. Having had some phenomenal teachers, instructors, professors, and mentors along the way has helped tremendously. In the not-too-distant past, nursing education was more punitive than supportive and nurturing. One instructor in my diploma program, whom I respected and was a little intimidated by, told me after an especially challenging student experience, "I don't know what it is about you, but you seem to know on a different level what you need to do. One of your two nurse aunts was a classmate of mine, and I remember she seemed to know just what to do, too. Because of this, I especially enjoy being your clinical supervisor." The positive feedback I received, and the validation that I was doing nursing right, made me think that maybe I could be an affirming teacher, and I might consider teaching nursing in the distant future.

Only five years later, my first opportunity came when I asked the dean and assistant dean in my baccalaureate program if they would write references for me for a staff position after I finished my nursing degree. Both flatly refused, saying that they had plans for me to enter the master's program, and they needed me to be an obstetric and pediatrics teaching assistant in the baccalaureate program that fall. I said I hadn't planned to start into a master's program that fall, but they were pretty convincing, so this became my newly revised plan.

Since the opportunity to teach presented itself before I had any formal preparation to teach, I tried very hard to learn on my own how to be a good teacher until I could take some courses in educational concepts. In my overcompensation to do well in this new role, I found I really enjoyed it, and students seemed to warm to my kind of teaching and responded favorably to our student-teacher interactions. To continue in nursing education, I was encouraged to get a doctorate in nursing, which I promptly did. All that I learned about teaching was to come in very handy as a nurse when patient teaching and lay education on health-related topics became paramount to quality nursing care and expected of every nurse. Again, I was at the right place at the right time to do the right thing as a teacher. I love being a teacher.

I have come full circle in my story of being a nurse, a mother, and a teacher. I'm grateful that I have been given the gifts of healing, helping, teaching, and I hope to continue to do so for many years to come. ♥

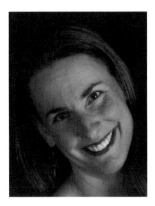

Marea Whitaker Bishop
Bellevue, NE
United States

**Phone** 402-981-7780

**E-mail**
openmindmarea@yahoo.com

www.photographybymarea.com

# Marea Whitaker Bishop

Marea lived in Europe from early childhood through her graduation from the University of Maryland in Heidelberg, Germany. Her passion for photography began during her teen years. Her father was an avid and accomplished photographer. Through observing him, she learned to recognize and compose appealing images from the architectural and cultural treasures at their doorstep.

She moved to Bellevue, Nebraska, in 1987, and seeks out all of the natural beauty to be found in this area, capturing it in her nature images.

*Photography by Marea* made its public debut in late 2002 and has since grown into a full service in-home Studio and Gallery. In 2008, Marea added destination photography to her menu of services, offering clients the option of her either accompanying families on their travels or meeting them at their holiday destinations for professional photo journaling of their once-in-a-lifetime adventures. She creates beautiful heirloom albums for them upon their return home.

# The Stages of Life

They say that a picture is worth a thousand words. A photograph that I took in August of 2000 has confirmed that adage many times over.

At the time, I was 36; my children were 4 and 5, and my husband and I had been married for 13 years. Our marriage appeared, from the outside, to be a better than average relationship, but underneath the surface there was discontent on both sides. We never fought; we seldom even argued. But I had not turned out to be the kind of wife he wanted, and I longed for a spiritual partnership in which personal growth would be encouraged and celebrated, which was not his "scene." Though we both adored our children and functioned together in our mutual love for them, in our own relationship we drifted even further apart.

I had struggled with depression on and off throughout our marriage. Through various therapies, I unearthed childhood abuse issues that had long been buried. I did my best to do the work, read the books, and process it all in order to put it behind me as expediently as possible; however, there is no express lane when it comes to *doing* healing work. At some point, my therapist recommended creative expression.

I tried to journal, but was never very consistent with it. I tried to paint, but felt my work was too elementary – like that of a young child. I judged my painting rather than understanding that the purpose of this process was about re-connecting with my inner creative self. Eventually, I picked up my camera and headed into nature, specifically, to a nearby forest trail that I had never hiked in summer before. When I came upon the marsh, it took my breath away. It was covered with a floating blanket of lotus blossoms and their exquisitely beautiful leaves. I was mesmerized. I had never seen anything like it. Time seemed to stand still as I shot an entire roll of film, then another. I was completely captivated by their beauty!

The following week, my mother-in-law called from Oklahoma, where she and my father-in-law were visiting their other grandchildren, and suggested that I bring our kids and take a weekend for myself. It was an unexpected and welcome offer, yet I could not think of where to go. I felt called by water, but the California coast, which was the first place that came to mind, was too far for just a three-day getaway. My in-laws ended up finding a Bed and Breakfast online just three hours south of where they were, at the edge of a national recreation area. I spoke with the owner, who happened to be a psychologist, and learned that she and her partner had purchased this facility as a place to host women's retreats. How perfect! My own private retreat house was waiting for me, complete with a massage therapist on standby. The Universe was providing me with a weekend of respite and casual counseling thrown in at no extra charge.

Just a few months before this weekend, I had begun working with a personal trainer in my neighborhood. On multiple occasions, we discovered that we both had been collecting quotes from a source identified as Abraham Hicks. Neither of us knew who this person was and just prior to my leaving on this trip to Oklahoma, my trainer googled the name and printed out a large stack of pages for me to take along for reading in my solitude. I packed them along with the two rolls of film I'd just had developed to look at once I got to my destination. The next day, I shared the photographic images with my hostess. I told her I had a sense that some of them were significant, but that I did not yet know why. One in particular stood out. It captured four different phases of the blooming process: the tight bud, the blossom just opening, full bloom, and the naked seed pod. It stirred something deep inside me.

My first evening at the B & B, I enjoyed an animated dinner with friends of my hosts. The second day, I was taken out in a row boat in the recreation area, then left to explore and stroll around the whole lake and find my way back to the inn later in the day. I spent that evening journaling. On my last day, I made myself comfortable in the hammock with my sheaf of Abraham Hicks reading material. This was my introduction to the Law of Attraction. I had never heard of it before, yet it resonated instantaneously with me. At once, I understood why so much in my life had seemed wrong for so long. All I knew how to do was focus on what

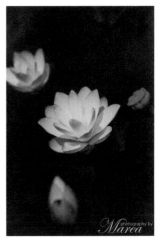

*The Four Stages of Life*

was wrong. I had never learned nor thought to do otherwise. I was filled with excitement and couldn't wait to get home to share this new information with my husband.

I clearly remember the conversation we had when I got home, in the back yard, just at the edge of our deck. I was practically bursting with enthusiasm for my new-found knowledge and how it would positively affect our relationship. I exclaimed, "I know what we've been doing wrong! We've been focusing on everything that is wrong with our marriage instead of focusing on what is *right*. All we have to do is make this shift and we can be happy again!" Nothing in the world could have prepared me for his response. Unbeknownst to me, while I was away opening heart and mind to Universal guidance, he was doing his own soul searching and had made the decision to leave. The ground fell out from under me. He gave me hope initially, suggesting it be a trial separation, but a year later he filed for divorce.

The following summer, I returned to the marsh to photograph the lotus again. This time it was a few weeks later in the season. I observed the seed pods in a fifth phase of the life cycle. They had turned brown and brittle, falling face first into the muddy waters as their delicate necks weakened and bent. The bumps on their little alien heads opening to reveal marble-sized seeds which would plant themselves in the wet earth when each pod surrendered itself to the "muck." I was blown away by the metaphor in this! Only in allowing the death of these once beautiful blossoms, in accepting the end, could new beginnings emerge. I saw, for the first time, beauty in something "dead," realizing that it is simply part of the process, the journey.

Fast forward to August 1, 2002: my children were away for the first time on a "family holiday" without me. I knew it could be torture to be by myself if I allowed it, or, I could make something positive of it. I promised myself to do one thing each day that I would not normally do. On this day, I went to the botanical gardens. I spent an hour or two photographing flowers and dragonflies, offering occasionally to take pictures for a group of ladies who were clearly there to celebrate a special occasion together. Before they left, they asked me if my pictures were for sale. I said that I had never sold any, that they were mostly just for me – my soul work. They said they would like to be my first customers. Two months later they came to my home where I had enlarged and framed quite a collection of my favorite images, among them my "Stages of Life." They admired all of my work but mostly wanted to purchase unframed prints for their scrapbooks. This left me with a large inventory of matted and framed nature photography, which led me to approach the forest gift shop about consigning my items.

The next thing I knew, I had my first display and sale at the gift shop's annual holiday market. It was there that I shared my lotus image and story for the first time. I met a woman who was looking for a gift for a friend who had cancer. The bare seed pod was reminiscent of the bald head of one who has just come through chemo, a reminder to hold onto hope, that the cycle repeats itself and life renews itself. She opened my eyes to how many ways this image can be interpreted and how it can encourage people in different ways along their healing journey. That picture was just the first of many which I have taken to inspire love, joy, and hope. We are so abundantly blessed by the beauty in nature. It offers so much to us through metaphors if we will only take the time to observe and contemplate.

One single image flashed a preview of the stages that were to come in my own life. Two seemingly random events, a walk in the forest and an outing to the botanical gardens, steered me into my healing process and into the next chapter of my life. I took photography classes, joined the professional associations, and have been a self-employed photographer ever since. With my photography, I have helped others along their healing journeys, donating my time and art to many charitable organizations. I have volunteered through "Now I Lay Me Down To Sleep," doing bereavement photography for families who have lost babies, creating memories for them to honor the too-short lives and comforting the parents through their grief.

At this time, I feel I am wrapping up this round of seed pod re-germinating. The first half of my life has been spent experiencing, learning, healing and forgiving. Now, I am a bud once again, preparing to blossom more magnificently than ever before. May I be a blessing to all I encounter through this process and may I be a friend and guide to others as they travel the healing path into discovering and living their own divine purpose! ♥

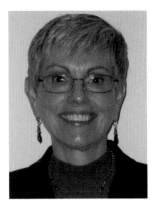

Dr. Mary Simon Leuci
Assistant Dean, College of
Agriculture Food and Natural
Resources
Program Director, Community
Development Extension
University of Missouri
232 Gentry Hall
Columbia, MO 65211
United States

**Phone** 573-882-2937

**E-mail** leucim@missouri.edu

http://extension.missouri.edu

# Dr. Mary Simon Leuci

In Mary's current role, she provides leadership for outreach programs statewide in community leadership development, community economic development, citizen engagement, community decision making, participatory planning, local government, creating inclusive communities, and community emergency management.

Mary is co-founder of the Community Development Academy and has also worked with communities and organizations to help develop Extension's VISTA program, community emergency management program, and others.

She currently serves on the North Central Regional Center for Rural Development Board. She also chairs the MU Provost's Quality of Life Committee as part of the Economic Development Initiative and is a 2009 national Food Systems Leadership Institute fellow.

Mary obtained her BS in Agriculture, MA in Adult Education, and EdD in Educational Leadership from the University of Missouri.

She has owned a greeting card business, enjoys gardening and cooking, volunteers her time at church, and spends most of her free time with her husband, Victor, and teenage daughter, Lena.

# Community is a Precious Gift

Christmas has always been a magical season that sparkles brightly for me. One memory stands out vividly: the December night was crisply cold, dark, and full of stars as we all gathered at the one-room Quisenberry School and piled into Dad's old truck – the one he used for hauling livestock, corn, soybeans, and anything else. He had placed a tarp over the top and sides to keep out the wind. On top was a freshly cut cedar tree encircled with big glowing colored Christmas lights. We were excited and chattered as 20 of us, ranging in ages seven to 18 years old, hopped aboard, bound in mittens, hats, coats, and boots. For the next two hours, Dad drove us around our rural "neighborhood" to homes and farmsteads of retirees, widows, and widowers. They were surprised and delighted to see this traveling marvel arrive! Margaret Arnett must have known we were coming because she had hot chocolate in Styrofoam cups waiting to warm our chilly bones. We sang and laughed our hearts out that night, but oh, the smiles and warmth we witnessed from our neighbors was priceless.

This was one of many 4-H activities that I participated in. (4-H is a youth development organization focused on leadership, citizenship, and life skills with the goal of making positive change.) My early ideas of developing community were formed in my Brown 4-H Club days. Our club's additional activities ranged from wildflower hikes and roadside clean-ups to the annual ice cream social with the Brown Ladies' Club. (Yes, it was all homemade – ice cream in black walnut, peach, and strawberry flavors plus many more, and delicious cakes and homemade blackberry cobbler. Yum!) There were Share-the-Fun nights when the clubs put on skits and plays. One year, one of my brothers and his friends dressed up like girls and were the characters in a skit. Another year, I was part of a Vaudeville act, being silly and laughing as we acted and sang. You need not worry – we also developed skills in knitting and sewing, electricity, woodworking, and leadership.

The other magical season? Easter, because it is God's life and love triumphant over death. In my first job, after graduating from college with my degree in agriculture, I worked in a wholesale greenhouse. I loved working with the plants and the soil, and nurturing new life as it connected me to God and his presence in nature. However, my new life was born in a church youth retreat during an Easter season just after completing college. I walked away knowing I was loved, that Christ was real. I understood to my very core that "I never walked alone," and that being in and building community was part of my spiritual journey.

Social justice and working for the common good have always been a part of who I am. This, too, came alive in 1980 when I jumped at the opportunity of a lifetime and spent four months in Sri Lanka living with families as an International 4-H Youth Exchangee (IFYE, and sometimes this stood for **I**'m the **F**ool **Y**ou **E**xpected, depending on the culture shock for the day!). When I moved in with my second host family after having been in the country only a few weeks, I was utterly overwhelmed by the 30 children who showed up nearly every day, sitting wherever they could in my family's small house, just to *be* with me. A family niece slept with me at night so I wouldn't be alone. I was often invited to dine at other homes in the village, and the entire Young Farmer's Club would show up to escort me as, clearly, they thought hosting me was part of their responsibility.

I was honored with village dance performances. The young men taught me how to play the drum with them. I am not exactly a gifted vocalist, but

I dug for my talents to share in return and sang the folk songs I had learned at 4-H club meetings. They loved every John Denver song I had memorized! After all, a gift from the heart and from one's own experience is worth more than any other. When I left that village, one young Buddhist in his late teens gave me a pencil drawing he had made for me. It was the Christian Nativity scene with characters that were clearly Sri Lankan. The drawing hangs framed in my home today.

I officially began my professional work in community development when I was 30, a few weeks before I walked down the aisle – first to wed my husband and second to receive my Master's degree. Sometimes I marvel at how I got here and what has kept me so engaged and so passionate about building community.

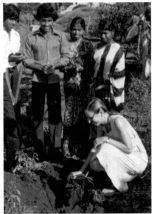

*I am planting a tree in Sri Lanka – a sign of friendship.*

One of my graduate school courses was a community development course taught by Jerry Wade, a professor and state community development extension specialist. I found excitement and satisfaction in the learning and work we did in the class. I was delighted when he asked after the semester, "If an opportunity comes along to work in community development extension with me, are you interested?" It was almost a year later when he called. I elatedly accepted and another key marker was staked in my journey. We were working with communities to help them dig out of the mid-1980s rural economic crisis.

It wasn't long before Jerry and I drove five hours to Ava, in rural southwest Missouri, as a winter storm approached. That evening, Jerry, Jack McCall (another community development colleague and mentor), and I were going to test a new "visioning" approach with a group of local citizens trying to grasp how they could improve the future for their community. We planned to ask several questions and facilitate a process for them to determine what they wanted the future to look like, and the steps they planned for launching their effort.

I vividly remember Jack phoning us from northwest Missouri saying he couldn't complete the trip due to the worsening winter storm. He said, "Mary, you can lead this." I told myself to use what skills and talents I had. When 30 people braved the freezing rain to work for three hours in large and small groups in the county court room that night, and then stayed to talk in a continued buzz, I knew something akin to magic had happened! The following summer when this community launched a watermelon festival to thank their volunteers, and later developed a leadership training program that included scholarships so they could include low-income citizens, I knew they had tapped the magic for themselves. I learned from Jack and Jerry, and others, "When they say, we did it ourselves, we know we have succeeded."

Twenty plus years have passed, and I am now the assistant dean that oversees the community development extension program. I have thrived on being part of innovative teams that work with communities to foster collaboration, improve rural health, seed alternative and new opportunities for small farmers, build inclusive communities, prepare and train for community emergency management, and create new economic opportunities. During all this time, I have seen the light bulbs go on as people say, "I just realized we have fought (amongst each other) all of our lives, but we really want the same things for our community." There is so much that I have learned from those who work to build and nurture and heal the community every day - whether they plan, organize, bake, tell stories, teach, lead, evaluate and reflect, *or* plant, water, weed, and harvest.

As it was then and is now, building community is about finding ways to challenge people to think and act differently – to innovate – to create vibrant local economies. The opportunities are ripe to bring people together in meaningful ways to listen to each other, determine how they can work together despite their differences, see things from new perspectives, repair broken bridges of relationship, and dream and build for the future.

Today, we hear so much about sustainability. For me, sustainability is and was rooted in seeing my Dad put in terraces and rotate crops before there was a sustainable agriculture movement. It is rooted in my living with families and spending time with nuns, Buddhists, Muslim women, and Hindus in Sri Lanka. From my humble, rural roots to living internationally in a very diverse setting, I learned that our communities are only sustainable if we engage our daughters and sons, our grandmothers and grandfathers, the unseen and the outspoken – all working for the common good and in the spirit of community well-being. The new challenges include passing the torch and helping the next generation – and the generation after that – see, understand, and continue to believe they can each make a difference, too.

I would know so much less about building community if it were not for Lena, my now teenage daughter. Her words, as a two-year old when I fastened her seat belt one day, will ever resound as a reminder of how we build community and, in the process, bring healing to our world: "Mommy, I am precious." Each and every person is precious and has a gift to give. Each and every community has unique gifts and resources with which to shape a collective future. We just have to stop, look, listen, respect, reflect, and share in order to recognize these gifts, nurture them, and bring them to fruition. I feel blessed to be able to play my part and help facilitate this for the world. ♥

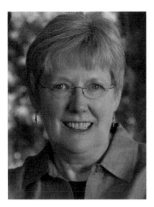

Barb Thune Schommer
348 Prior Avenue North
Suite #105
St Paul, MN 55104
United States

**Phone** 763-458-0220

**E-mail**
Barb.Schommer@gmail.com

# Barb Thune Schommer

Barb is a registered nurse. She came into healing and energy work midway through a 40-year career as a public health nurse. As a Certified Healing Touch Practitioner, she delights in bringing Healing Touch to people within her own private practice and to the community as a hospital volunteer. She is a frequent community speaker about energy healing. Barb believes in the restorative power within each of us and she enjoys assisting people in their own self-healing journey.

As a Certified Healing Touch Instructor, Barb is gentle and loving in her approach of allowing participants to unfold in their own life healing journey as they experience Healing Touch workshops.

Barb is a charter member of Healing Touch International.

# Wisdom Comes in Small Packages

I am a Certified Healing Touch Practitioner practicing in both my healing office and as a volunteer at a local hospital. I was drawn into attending my first Healing Touch class by answering a flyer that came in the mail. I believe we are guided in our lives to the work that can become a passion. It was that way for me. I took one class, and then others, and then became certified in this energy work for which I have a deep passion.

Healing Touch is a gentle way to calm, bring relaxation, and relieve pain, using a heart-centered approach to moving and clearing the energy field that is around each of us (commonly referred to as the aura or biofield). Clearing is done using the hands, which may or may not touch the person receiving the Healing Touch treatment. The goal in Healing Touch is to restore wholeness through harmony and balance, allowing the receiver to move into a place of self healing.

Through the years, I have been privileged to provide Healing Touch for many different people with a variety of health issues and in a variety of life situations. My learning continues as I work with clients like Anna, who brought deep personal growth and wisdom in a very small package.

I had given Healing Touch to Anna's mother several times throughout her first pregnancy and again late in her pregnancy with Anna. When I work with a pregnant woman, I connect with her, and ask her permission to also connect with her unborn child. The child's energy field extends beyond the physical body of the mother, and can be sensed by the practitioner. I sensed Anna's sweet loving energy when I connected with her. Anna's mother and I determined that she and I would work together to clear her field and facilitate her in coming into balance and harmony, as well as help move her into a relaxed place for her upcoming delivery.

Anna was born on September 29 and experienced four days at home with her Mom, Dad, and big brother. Her mom told me she had been born with an "uneven" heart beat, but that the doctors told them not to worry because it would correct itself. On the fifth day, Anna began nursing less and sleeping more, and her parents took her to the hospital where her heart was beating 260 to 300 beats a minute (which is extremely fast for a newborn, whose regular heart beat would be around 120 beats per minute). Anna was rushed into pediatric intensive care and her parents began a round-the-clock vigil with her.

I had been trying to call the parents around the time I thought Anna would be born, but had not reached them. They were overwhelmed by Anna's medical condition and forgot to contact me. When Anna's mom did call, Anna was about a month old and her mom told me of her hospitalization and numerous medical challenges. Anna's Mom asked me to come to the hospital to provide Healing Touch for Anna. I agreed and met Anna for the first time in the Pediatric Intensive Care unit of the hospital on November 3rd.

Anna was a full-term baby of normal weight and she looked healthy, except for her puffy face and all the tubes and ventilator and bells and alarms sounding frequently in her intensive care room. Already in her very short life, she had survived kidney failure, a massive infection, lung problems, liver failure, and a weak heart.

When I entered her room, I was struck by all the pictures of roses her parents had placed around her – taped to the bed, on the walls, on the frames that held all the tubes and medical equipment. It was a garden of beauty for a beautiful little girl. I walked up to Anna's bed gently, coming carefully into her field and assessing her response to my movement. She remained calm as I moved my hand over her field, and then I gently began clearing the congestion that I sensed was present over her entire field. My intention was to clear any congestion that was caused by all the medication and medical procedures she had undergone. The clearing would complement the medical care to maximize the benefits of all her other treatments.

Anna remained calm as I worked. I could see a tiny change in her face; the muscles around her small mouth relaxed a bit. She was in a coma, not opening her eyes, not moving any part of her body, and not making a sound. I completed our session when her field felt clear of the congestion I had sensed at first. As I prepared to leave, I held Anna's small hand and said a blessing for her and her parents. They were close by as I worked, and said after the treatment that they felt a sense of calm and had themselves become relaxed during the time I was working with Anna. It often happens that caregivers receive much-needed calming and relaxation during the treatment of someone they love.

I visited Anna every other day for the next week or so, always approaching her gently, watching for any sign that I was entering her field too fast. During our clearing sessions, Anna remained unresponsive, but did wiggle a bit at the end of one of our clearing sessions. My sense was that she had had enough Healing Touch for the day.

One day when I arrived at the hospital, I learned one of the procedures that was being tried for Anna's kidney failure was not working. The medical team had decided to try using regular dialysis through the blood system. During this Healing Touch session, I worked over her abdomen, clearing and moving congestion from this area. By the time I was done, her field was clear and she was breathing more slowly. The ever-present monitors also showed a slowing of her heart beat, slowing of her respirations, and an increase in her blood oxygen levels. According to the monitors, she was becoming relaxed.

It was mid-November when Anna's Mom contacted me telling me Anna was not improving and was, in fact, experiencing additional organ failure. The medical team was out of options and ideas. When I arrived to visit Anna that day, there was a heaviness about her. Her skin was pale yellow with the onset of liver failure. She continued to be in a coma. Even though her Mom and Dad had been constantly at her side, stroking her, talking softly with her, holding her hand, she was completely non-responsive to any kind of stimulus.

When I worked with Anna that day, I used a Healing Touch intervention called the Chakra Spread, which is very helpful during times of transition. I sensed that Anna was going through a huge life transition at this time. As I did the Chakra Spread with her, I sensed the heaviness lifting. When I held her hand and hovered my other hand over her heart, I sensed a remarkable peace and calm flooding through me and through Anna. Anna's parents who were in the room also sensed the tremendous peace and calm. Perhaps the Chakra Spread gave all of them – Anna and her parents – the space and love they needed for this parting.

Feeling this peace helped them make the difficult decision to discontinue life support (a decision they had been talking about with the medical team for the past few days but had not been able to finalize). Now, Anna was able to die in their arms without any tubes or a ventilator. In her last moments, she opened an eye, looked at them and moved her head to nurse at her Mom's breast. This was a difficult transition for her parents, but also one they now talk about as being so loving, peaceful, and calm.

I am honored that Anna and her parents allowed me to be a part of their life journey. Although Anna and I worked together only a short time, she had a profound impact on me. She taught me to trust my intuitive nature by listening to her non-verbal communication. She taught me the profound nature of unconditional love as I watched her parents care for her and as they allowed me to join them in that caring. She allowed me to walk with her on her life journey and to touch her wisdom. By her life and her death she shared the circle of life with me. Yes, wisdom does come in small packages. My heart is filled with gratitude for you, Anna! ♥

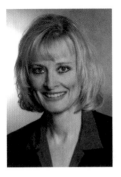

Mary Beth Lamb
4100 Cedar Lake Rd.
St. Louis Park, MN 55416
United States

**Phone** 952-925-4002

**E-mail** mblamb@q.com

# Mary Beth Lamb

Mary Beth has helped business people in more than 20 industries on five continents achieve peak performance and maximize return on worldwide business investment by developing cultural competency. She coaches, consults, facilitates and speaks worldwide on global leadership, multicultural sales and service effectiveness, virtual teamwork, global diversity, and knowledge transfer across cultures.

In 1998, Wilson Learning Worldwide acquired the intercultural training company she co-founded in 1991, *Transnational Strategies, Inc.*

Lamb also co-authored the critically acclaimed book *Do's and Taboos Around the World for Women in Business.* She is writing a second book on leveraging virtual, multicultural teams.

Mary Beth is married and has three children: Lucas, Nathan and Emma.

# A Chinese Lesson in Global Healing

Empathy. The ability to put yourself in someone else's shoes. That's a trait highly valued in people whose work requires them to span time, space, cultures, and organizations.

Whether it's our neighbor at the bus stop, the customer service rep on the phone, or our coworker in the next cubicle, all of us need empathy to help us recognize and bridge cultural differences that impact how we think, act, communicate, and, perhaps most critically, motivate people differently across cultures.

For almost 20 years it has been my passion to work as a cross-cultural facilitator, speaker, and consultant. I work with groups and individuals at corporations, universities, and schools to build empathy and trust by helping people identify and learn to appreciate differences that impact their work and lives.

Once we *recognize* those differences, we can use empathy, emotional intelligence, and other practical tools to capitalize on those differences.

And now for the real truth: For me this work is also about building fragile boards toward each other in a global suspension bridge of peace. It's about healing those who have suffered or been frightened when confronted with differences they didn't understand. It's about healing those who have been discriminated against or marginalized because of differences that others did not see or accept. Often these misunderstandings cause frustration and pain. Sometimes they lead to war and destruction.

So how are we to address such a risky cultural divide? One way is to work with functioning global institutions that already span these differences. In that regard, I see myself as a kind of intercultural guerrilla. Facilitating world peace may not be the main reason I'm hired, but it can always be one of the outcomes, if the participants so choose.

Recently this work took me to China to train some Chinese consultants to do similar cross-cultural work across Asia. It was on this trip that I learned what empathy *really* means.

My lesson began with the moment we fear our whole lives. While I was in Shanghai, more than 7,000 miles from home, I learned that my mother was dying. I had to get home.

But I was at a loss. How do you convey your anguish, guilt, and panic to near strangers, people with very different worldviews, colleagues whom you've known for less than a week? How do you convey loss without breaking down in front of your new peers?

There was no time for internal constipation. I grabbed the first person I could find and closed the door behind us. To my dismay and his, I immediately broke down into tears. This sophisticated Beijing man did not know what to do or say. I knew he wanted to be anyplace in the world other than here with me.

Empathy! He must have thought of it. For in what must have been for him a gut-wrenching moment, he slowly and gingerly reached out his hand toward me, ever so lightly he patted my hand and said, "I'll get you tea." And then he fled.

The next person to enter the room had spent seven years in the United States so he knew what it meant to cross cultures at work and home. He'd had a lot of practice building empathy because he truly saw life through both Chinese and U.S. eyes. That's how he knew that Americans liked to be told, "Everything will be okay," even if it won't be. So that's what he told me. Then he, too, quickly exited.

The final visitor was a Hong Kong native who'd spent half his life in Canada. His North American-style empathy was almost at the subconscious level. As he walked toward me, arms open wide, I knew I would get the bear hug I most craved at that moment. And my crying? No problem. He encouraged it and got me more tissues.

I've described three different faces of empathy. Whose gesture had the most impact? For me it was the first man, for even while he was gathering up his courage to touch my hand, part of me was viewing our interaction as would a fly on the wall. And as I both watched and participated in our exchange, I felt amazed and grateful. For him that simple hand pat was like an emotional leap across the Great Wall of China. He adapted far outside his comfort zone to meet my needs. Even today I cannot truly fathom it.

When I finally stopped hiccupping, I wiped my eyes and opened the conference room door. To my surprise I found that everyone in the entire office had stopped work to help me.

Seemingly without overt direction or even a verbal exchange, each person in that office was now working feverishly to get me home as quickly as possible. Some were quietly packing my training supplies, others were bringing me refreshments, two more were working the phones to find me an earlier flight home. Before they gently scooted me into the waiting taxi though, there was one cultural norm that could not be violated.

We had to take a final group picture of us all, smiling. And just then I understood something fundamental about my Chinese friends. The Chinese say that life is suffering. For most of us westerners that seems so, well, negative.

But perhaps this realistic worldview is not so negative if we reframe it as the Chinese may see it. For there is suffering in life. But for them, it is suffering with others; they draw solace by knowing that the work team, the family, and the community will always be there for you during the hard times. Perhaps that makes the suffering more bearable because you are not alone, and through the wisdom of the group there can be new growth, new learning.

**So that day the teacher became the student. And the healer became the healed.**

And I learned that healing the world is not as idealistic or subversive as I had once thought, but rather something we can *each* do. It may be as simple as taking a deep breath, opening our scarred hearts a crack, and extending our hand in the universally understood gesture that means, "Help me, please."

And when that help comes, fearfully, fleetingly, or wrapped in a bear hug, let's cherish that moment and vow to do the same for the next person who reaches out for our help. ♥

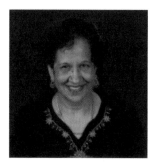

Dr. Shashi Sharma
12114 Linden Lane
Overland Park, KS 66209
United States

**Phone** 785-342-1899

**E-mail** shashispirit@gmail.com

# Dr. Shashi Sharma

Shashi is a board certified pediatrician who has worked with children and their families for more than 30 years. She has been a part of international medical mission tours, including countries such as the Dominican Republic, Guatemala, Honduras, and India. Her current goal is to work in India, establishing a non-profit clinic for the welfare of underserved children and elderly, and also to run a mobile medical clinic for remote areas in Rajasthan, India.

# Here Comes That Negro Doctor!

It was a normal afternoon in a pediatric office of a Midwest rural community with a population of approximately 40,000 people. I had resided in this small town for about five years, and had lived in the Midwest for twice as long. The town contained a small nursing college, and a remote campus of technology and state university students. Most of the people living in town were Caucasian, with a small blend of African Americans, Mexican Americans, and various small immigrant populations from Vietnam, Japan, and a family or two from China. I happened to be one of two female pediatricians in town, but the only female pediatrician from India.

I loved living in a small town. I loved the "easy access" to almost everything without waiting in long lines or having to drive twenty minutes in bumper-to-bumper traffic just to go from point A to point B, as often happens in a big city. I thoroughly enjoyed practicing medicine in this small town, as well. I got to know my patients and their families on a whole new level because not only did they receive continuity of care in my examination room, but they might also be my neighbors. I loved being greeted wherever I went with happy yells of, "Hello, Dr. Sharma!" accompanied with a big smile and a hug.

My afternoon clinic sessions usually started around 1:30 p.m. I was about to encounter my first patient for the afternoon. As I entered the room, I heard a young voice exclaim, "Here comes that Negro doctor!" I smiled and looked at the family sitting in front of me; Mom and Dad were sitting on the guest chairs, the younger brother on Mom's lap, and a handsome "little man" was sitting proudly on the exam table.

While having practiced medicine in the United States for more than 18 years by that time, I was taken aback with the comment from an innocent 10 year-old boy. It was the first time I was greeted as a "Negro doctor," instead of being welcomed with greetings such as, "Hola!" "Hi doc!" or "Namaste." I smiled, while the boy's mom blushed and his dad frowned at him. My young patient and I made eye contact and I extended my hand. I introduced myself, "Hi there! I'm Dr. Sharma. Are you Dave?" He hesitantly took my hand in his and smiled sheepishly, wondering what he had said wrong as he looked at the facial expressions of his parents. To break the ice I said, "Dave, I will give you a dollar if you can guess correctly the country of my origin, since I am not African American." For a few seconds, Dave seemed lost deep in thought. Suddenly, as if a light bulb went off, he piped up with an answer, "You are from Mexico!" I shook my head "no," and he exclaimed, "You are from China!" Obviously he lost the dollar, but he gained an instant friend!

As the years went by, Dave came to visit me often, not only for his needed doctor visits but just to talk. I answered his curious mind's questions whenever I could. Unfortunately, when he was in high school, like many teenagers Dave's curiosity got the best of him and he became involved with a group of at-risk teenagers who were using drugs and engaging in high-risk behavior. Naturally concerned for his son, Dave's father made an appointment for the two of them to see me.

Being a primary care provider and my patient's advocate, I always ask my patient if they want their parents in the room when they talk to me or when I examine them. (Their privacy and comfort are my concern, especially when they are teenagers.) Dave requested that his father not be present when he talked with me.

Dave, who looked quite stressed and tired, began our visit by telling me how "messed up" he felt. He told me his friends had encouraged him to start drinking. At first, it was only a beer here and there, but it had become a regular after-school activity. He denied smoking cigarettes or any other "funny stuff," as well as the use of any other drugs. His friends, though, were experimenting with "weed" at that time. School was becoming difficult for him, as he was getting into trouble and had been getting into physical fights with other students. Home life wasn't any easier for Dave. He was increasingly getting into arguments with his parents.

We talked about addiction and the toll it took on individuals, and, like most teenagers who "know it all," he knew what alcohol could do to a young, healthy body. Since he did not want to visit a "shrink" and was comfortable talking to me, we left the conversation with a promise of him returning to my office within a week to continue our dialogue. I was deeply concerned about him and I was relieved he felt comfortable enough to talk about his feelings and did not feel judged by me.

A week later, Dave did not show up as promised, but his mom did. Dave's mom was a nice, soft spoken lady who seemed to be the "mediator" of her family and who continuously lost out to two very stubborn males in her household. She showed up in my office deeply upset and crying. She began to tell me that she felt "hopeless," that Dave had not been coming home at night, was flunking out of school, and had become increasingly violent and threatening towards her. She was scared for both him and herself. She continued explaining to me that Dave's father worked very long hours, and the times when he and Dave were home together, they would have huge, blowout arguments. At one point she mentioned that Dave had "his father's genes" and she was incapable of stopping either one of them when they argued.

I strongly recommended that they go immediately into family counseling. However, Dave's mom was very uncertain that either her husband or her son would go for psychological or psychiatric help. Instead, she thought they would be more willing to come to me. (In my mind, I imagined a scene at their dinner table, where she was begging both Dave and his father to get some help and try to solve their on-going problems, but her cries fell upon deaf ears.)

Dave and his dad never showed up in my office. It was a long time after that when I saw Dave, now a handsome young man, on a summer afternoon in our town mall. He was paired up with a pretty young girl. We waved at each other from a distance and, as I got closer, I realized his young girlfriend was also a patient of mine. We all had a brief, friendly exchange of greetings and went our separate ways. I secretly hoped that Dave would come and visit me again.

A few weeks later, he did. He came to see me because he "didn't know where else to go." He was heartbroken because his girlfriend had broken up with him since he didn't comply with all of her demands. During this visit he confessed that he had a short temper and, to express his anger, he would hit walls and throw furniture. He again expressed he did not want to see a psychologist or psychiatrist, but would do whatever I thought would be best for him. He agreed to take medication if he had to – what a breakthrough! I was honored that he entrusted me with his feelings and that he knew I had his best interest at heart and would provide him with the best medical care in my capacity. Together, we devised a plan of healthier relationships and living for Dave.

As a pediatrician, one is sometimes lucky enough to watch your patients grow up to the age of 18. When Dave turned 18, he and his father asked if it would be okay to continue to visit me. I continued to see Dave whenever he wanted until I left my practice 10 years later. During one of those rare visits, he mentioned casually about possibly joining the Army.

I will never forget the first day I met Dave, with his reservations and pre-conceived notions of me being "that Negro doctor," and what I did in those few minutes in that initial encounter to gain his unbridled trust and friendship. I often think of Dave and wonder about him. Did he join the Army? Did he get deployed to Iraq? Is he alive? How is his family doing? Did he find new love and build a family of his own?

I guess the "take home" message here is that humanity encompasses many colors. A color alone is pretty enough, but a bunch of colors together with understanding and trust sure makes one heck of a beautiful human rainbow! ♥

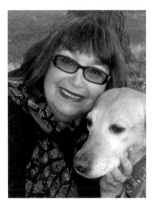

Connie Nelson Ahlberg
12713 Welcome Lane
Burnsville, MN 55337
United States

**Phone** 952-894-5008

**E-mail** cjnapoet@comcast.net

# Connie Nelson Ahlberg

Connie was born in Duluth, Minnesota with strong family roots on the North Shore of Lake Superior in Lutsen (where great-grandparents, C.A. and Anna Nelson, started Lutsen Resort before the turn of the century). A former educator of 10 years, she turned writer in the fall of 1986. Profoundly spiritual, she has written prayers in prose for those both in and out of recovery or "discovery." In addition, she has either written a thought, or can compose one on the spot: on loss, love, family, or friendship. She looks for sacredness and truth in everyday life, drawing from her Christian roots, as well as the mindfulness of Zen. Her prose honors in unique ways – and is written with family and friends as her source of inspiration. In the 1990s, she dressed words in ribbons and sold them in hospitals, gift shops, and boutiques throughout the state of Minnesota and beyond. Connie is currently writing about loss and healing. She lives in Burnsville, Minnesota, with her dog, Courage.

# Love within Life

Many faiths say we are all called to be healers.

I think the seeds, the spiritual links of body, mind, heart, and hope, are in the marrow of our bones from childhood. I once asked, "Why does God want me to catch all these fish?" following a family fishing event. Even at that tender age of five, I was a seeker on a quest of deeper understanding. This continued at my first school experience at the Cathedral of Our Lady of the Rosary in Duluth, Minnesota. It overlooked that giant – Lake Superior. Now almost six decades later, I realize every woman can be a part of a rosary of caring in the world – a giving bead, a healing bead – a prayer to lift the world.

My passage to become a prayer came not only from the richness of my path, but also the pain felt through hardship which honed my heart. While many battle different diseases, for me life's challenges knocked at my door in the form of depression. But it not only knocked, it moved right in. And this unwanted visitor was like a house guest that doesn't know when to leave. I would learn much later that my disease was passed on to me like a baton in an Olympic relay race: "Got it? GO!" I went!

Later, despite every dream, my relationships floundered; and jobs seemed too arduous in the harsh light of day. I became acutely aware that I was vulnerable in the swirl of loss. With depression, the symptoms of the disease take over. It is then you have to learn how to live with both your problems and this imbalance that whispers in your ear: You might as well quit.

NO. I chose to educate myself about the symptoms of this disease. At a visceral level, I "got" that pain and loss offer an opportunity to *transcend* in body and spirit what I had been saying "yes" to on a soul level for years. I penned, "Loss offers the most transformative path for our evolution."

After honoring a former teacher and mentor in a tribute, I was asked, "Have you ever thought about writing?" Thus, the desire to lift others with my prose became my path. As one deepens, you comprehend the suffering in others. I realized then my own redemption would rise like Spirit above the Self. It is like taking the compost of our pain and from it, rising like a Phoenix. From this journey, not always chosen, I share what's been given to me – a wand of weaving words. I have come to more fully understand what I wrote years ago:

Those who have known
Grief, loss or despair--
And continue to rise above it,
Show the resiliency
Of the human spirit;
And the God within.

Depression is my "Achilles Heel." I do well and – without warning – as I process a loss or a family event I can slip into the depths of darkness. Yet, the problems of life are *solved by life*. The very problem you may not want to face can only be dealt with by grabbing it around the neck! As American Buddhist nun, Pema Chodron, and other Buddhists teach: "Lean into it."

Lean into adversity. Go into the cave with your monsters. Stare them down. Even though the snake slithers towards you, get busy leaning into what you face. When you wake in the morning, the demons are gone. It is just you in the cave.

We never *arrive*. And we can't rest on our laurels. Groundlessness is just around the corner. No, it is under our feet! This moment is all we have. We are here to evolve – to ease the suffering of the world. I believe we are here to live in loving-kindness, compassion, and integrity. We are here to serve.

On this journey, perhaps I've given birth to twins: Prayer and Loss. It is near impossible to separate the two. Loss has been my transformation, just as prayer became my plea and healer. It's as if loss is my canoe, and healing prayer the water of my salvation. Once washed by Grace in wave upon wave – you seek to be a conduit through healing prayer for others.

My words are the Grace in my Baptism. Words are the mouth of my river. My prose is God's gifts I was meant to share. Friends say I have a direct line to the Divine. In truth, I don't know where my words come from. I believe they come from outside me.

God really listens when we ask in the name of those we care about, rather than for ourselves. And so my poetic words are about others; I write to honor you. I see the Light in your eyes, the strength in your *soul*, the beauty in *your* gifts and…I am in awe!

If we didn't experience loss, we couldn't deepen, and it is in deepening that I know what pain is. It is my pain that awakens me to see yours and seeks to reach out – to you. As I wrote in 1996:

Our personal stories of loss are really our stories of love;
If we hadn't had our years of love and bonding,
If the riches weren't there, how could our tears fall
Over our warmed hearts?
Truly loss is a circle of love within life.

Women soften the world; we have the hands and heart. Our souls applaud each other! To all women I say let us go as Grace; let us be beads on a rosary of prayers in the world. I honor you with words written in1994 in my poem called "Women are Perennials."

Women are perennials
Starting out
As little green shoots;
Then to annuals, the hardest stage,

Uprooted time after time;
Until they become hostas
With wide skirts and tall purple blossoms;
And when they gather,
In grace and dignity
Wide leaves touching,
There is nothing
As beautiful – as they. ♥

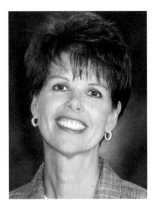

Cindy Bultena
*Woodwinds Health Campus*
1925 Woodwinds Dr.
Woodbury, MN 55125
United States

**Phone** 651-232-0100

**E-mail** cbultena@healtheast.org

www.woodwinds.org

# Cindy Bultena

Prior to joining the Woodwinds team, Cindy served in a variety of hospital administrative positions, including Assistant Director of Nursing, Medical Surgical Educator, Home Care Coordinator and Associate Administrator of Patient Care Services.

As the Executive Lead for Healing and Clinical Coordination at *Woodwinds Health Campus*, Cindy is instrumental in the creation and integration of a holistic patient and family-centered care model for a 78-bed inpatient hospital that opened in August 2000. She continues to serve on the Leadership Team to evolve Woodwinds' Vision and Guiding Principles.

Cindy holds an AA degree in Nursing from Rochester Community College and a BS degree in Community Health from Mankato State University, both in Minnesota. She also holds an MS degree in Nursing Administration from the University of Minnesota.

# Three Angels on a T-Shirt

One of the things I had planned for a vacation in Florida in March 1997 was to decide whether to apply for an exciting position helping to design a new hospital called Woodwinds Health Campus in Woodbury, Minnesota. This would be a huge stretch for me, and I just wasn't sure I had what was needed to make this project succeed. While in a souvenir shop one day, I saw a t-shirt...

On the front of the shirt were three colorful angels and a poem: "Your angels are there in your time of need, not to question or judge but to give you a lead. It may be a vision or a voice you hear, they just want to tell you that magic is near. So pick yourself up and go after your dream, you will never have a better home team."

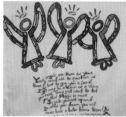

*My angel T-shirt*

I considered this to be my message from God that I was to apply for the job. When I returned home, I called Julie Schmidt, CEO of Woodwinds, to set up an interview. On July 7, 1997 I began my role as the Executive Lead of Healing and Clinical Coordination for Woodwinds Hospital.

Seeing that T-shirt transformed my career and, in many ways, my life. For the next three years, I was part of a three-woman design team that was formed to build this new hospital. The vision of Woodwinds was, "To be tne innovative, unique, and preferred resource for health by fundamentally creating the healthcare experience in a way that had not been done before." The community had articulated their vision of healthcare in the 21st century – and we were the team to help make it happen.

For the past nine years, I have been a part of the senior leadership team at Woodwinds to actualize our vision. For me to tell my personal story, I need to describe what this hospital is like.

Built on a holistic framework of body, mind, and spirit, Woodwinds' healing environment provides a natural and home-like experience with evidence-based selection of colors, fabrics, lighting, wood, curves, and access to views of nature. This environment is key to healing for patients and staff alike. The Model of Care integrates the use of healing arts into the scope of nursing care. This includes energy medicine (Healing Touch and Reiki), essential oils, guided imagery, acupuncture, and music therapy. These therapies create the ultimate patient experience. Further, our employees know that although they cannot always take advantage of the healing arts, they are there to support their individual self-care plans. Because employees value and nurture a healing and healthy relationship with themselves, they are able to care for their patients and others in the spirit of compassionate service.

We have worked hard to create a corporate culture and a healing space for our staff to be at their best. The "fruits of our labor" show in the following results:

- Woodwinds recently received the "Best Hospital Workplace" Award from the Minnesota Hospital Association.
- Patient satisfaction at Woodwinds is in the 92nd percentile in the United States and, at times, the obstetric satisfaction scores at Woodwinds have been the highest in the country.
- Nursing engagement (similar to a satisfaction score), as measured by the Gallup Poll, has also been the highest of any hospital in the U.S.
- HealthEast, the hospital system that Woodwinds is a part of, was just

recognized as being one of the top 10 hospital systems in the country for clinical excellence.

From the beginning, our management team incorporated the principles of servant leadership into our work to bring the values of compassionate service alive. Julie frequently reminded us, "Our work is about helping each and every employee – to *be* who they are."

Even in my initial interview, this "be who you are" philosophy struck a deep chord within me. All of a sudden I felt like my career and life "came together"…it all made sense. It was as if I had been preparing for this moment for the past twenty years! These powerful words resonated with me – freed me from the "shoulds" I had been feeling, and raised the expectation for me to be my best. As I moved more and more into my leadership role at Woodwinds, I found new solutions to old problems through increased creativity. I was willing to take more risks, and I listened to my intuition. This led me to have much more confidence in myself and others. I was recreating my role as a leader and it felt great!

My goal is to live the vision and values each day. As I model this to those I coach and serve, they are encouraged to serve our patients and each other with their best.

I view leadership as a call to greatness – both at work and at home. Several years ago, I wrote my own personal mission statement, "compassionate service to my self, family and community." Only since my experience at Woodwinds have I really paid attention and intention to what that means in my life. First, it is about being the best for me, and then for those closest to me (my family and friends), and, ultimately, for the community/world. Serving others is really why I am on this earth. That clarity brings a strong sense of direction and purpose for me.

Each month we greet new employees at Woodwinds and we invite our leaders to share why they picked Woodwinds. Many have their own versions of the role God played in their destiny. For me, I like to tell the story of a special T- shirt…I still have it and I always will! ♥

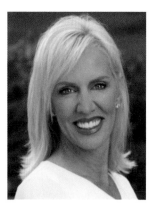

Kay Casperson
*Inside by Kay Casperson*
2402 Palm Ridge Road
Unit 2-111
Sanibel, FL 33957
United States

**Phone** 239-404-4848

**E-mail** kay@kaycasperson.com

www.kaycasperson.com

# Kay Casperson

Kay has worked for more than 25 years in many aspects of the beauty industry, from consulting, teaching and training, to researching and developing beauty products. Her life's work has led her to become a nationally recognized beauty and lifestyle expert, sharing her tips, tools and techniques for becoming a more beautiful person inside and out, and ultimately helping others to create true success and happiness in their lives.

Kay is expanding her retail stores and representatives nationally and has plans for a multi-media outreach that will continue to bring the message of "beauty inside out" to the world. She resides on Sanibel Island with her husband, Trevor, and two beautiful daughters, Kayla and Kayce, where she experiences the lifestyle that she promotes every day.

# Beauty with a Purpose

I feel blessed to have found my purpose at a very young age...or maybe I was just following my heart!

As a little girl and then as a teenager and into adulthood, I always had a passion to help other girls feel better about themselves. I remember being a good listener to people's needs and finding a solution to help them be better or at least feel better. Even as a young girl I remember helping my friends with their hair and makeup and dressing them up, and getting so much satisfaction from seeing a smile on their face!

In my life journey, I have met many people who had what the world would define as physical beauty, but they could hardly even look in the mirror without criticizing themselves and talking about their flaws. On the flip side, I also met people who would walk into a room and shine with beauty that was "bubbling over" from within. Yet, they could not pull it all together on the outside and, therefore, did not have the complete confidence to accomplish everything they wanted.

To me, beauty is everywhere and in everyone...sometimes, still waiting to be discovered! After searching for the *real* meaning of the word "beauty," I learned many years ago that you can't find this in a jar of cream, a lipstick tube, or in the pages of a magazine. *Real beauty* is something that has to come from within. As this became clearer to me, I also realized this meant living life balanced in five areas: 1) emotional (your thoughts and feelings), 2) spiritual (deeply held beliefs), 3) physical (your body), 4) environmental (your surroundings), and, 5) social (the people who are allowed into your life). When we keep these areas in balance, we discover *true beauty*.

This is the foundation of the lifestyle I developed called *Beauty Inside Out*. My goal is to help people discover what is inside and, at the same time, help them find balance on the outside. I have learned that this is not a sudden transformation, but a gentle evolution.

What was going to be my tool to help in this evolutionary process? After being involved in the beauty industry for many years in various capacities including consulting, teaching, and training, as well as researching and developing beauty products, I decided to create beauty enhancement products and incorporate heart-felt messages on each of the products.

I began by putting affirmations and positive statements on my product lines – skincare, hair care, cosmetics, and accessories. The purpose was two-fold: helping people maintain physical beauty while reminding them how to stay balanced. For example, my core skincare line consists of six products:

- *Remove* is the cleanser. On the back of the bottle is the statement, "identify and remove negative influences in your life."
- *Refresh*, the toner, has a statement to, "introduce positive alternatives to the things that you have removed."
- *Repair,* which is a healing gel, says, "address problems that might require a long-term commitment." (Examples could include forgiving others, healing relationships, etc.).
- *Revitalize* stimulates collagen production, keeping our skin looking young. The affirmation is, "I will bring vitality to my life."
- *Replenish* is a moisturizer with the loving thought, "I will take time to care for myself."
- *Renew* minimizes the appearance of fine lines and wrinkles. The thought for this step of the process is, "I will decide what I want for my future and set goals."

As I travel around the country, I see women (and men) using these simple products and really taking the messages to heart, developing confidence and making changes both internally and externally. Their stories of healing – of transformation – are amazing.

Over 25 years ago, my mission was to help people find the delicate balance between inner and outer beauty, and how vital it is for happiness to have both. Today, my product line expansions still center on this important inspirational message: "Take care of your life, as well as your physical body." This is, indeed, healing that the world needs. ♥

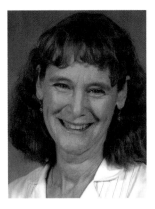

Helen Wells O'Brien
*Regions Hospital*
640 Jackson St.
St. Paul, MN 55101
United States

**Phone** 651-254-1363

**E-mail** Helen.W.Obrien@
HealthPartners.com

# Helen Wells O'Brien

Helen has served as a staff chaplain since 1998 for *Regions Hospital* and *Gillette Children's Specialty Healthcare* in St. Paul, Minnesota. Her work as a chaplain focuses primarily on pediatric patients who have experienced traumatic injury – including brain, spinal cord and burn injuries – and their families. Her work at Gillette also includes serving children, teens, and adults in the disability community. She chairs Gillette's ethics committee and is a member of the Gillette palliative care team.

Helen is the author of *Out of Ashes* (Herald Press, 1991). She is an ordained Mennonite minister. She has a Master's of Education degree with a specialty in reading disabilities, and taught in the Chaska, Minnesota, public schools (1976-1980) and at Red School House in St. Paul (1981-1982).

Helen has two adult sons, Joseph and Daniel Wells Quintela. Her favorite things are hiking, bicycling, canoeing, traveling with husband John, and working in her garden.

# Keeping the Watch:
# The Life of a Hospital Chaplain

Mark was a young member of the St. Paul Mennonite Fellowship, a small congregation in St. Paul, Minnesota, where I served as pastor for 12 years. He was born prematurely at 24 weeks and survived. At age six, Mark was diagnosed with a malignant brain tumor. His year-long journey with a devastating disease would transform our church family. Our active urban community church was essentially called upon to *be still* and to accompany our littlest and most beloved member as he died.

It was a year in which we sang, cried, laughed, carried, cooked, and took turns providing respite care. It was also when I began to ponder the whole meaning of faith, healing, and community. I learned that there was nothing I could do – nothing that any of us could do – to change the course of Mark's dying. The only power we had was to be fully present for the remainder of his precious days with us. And so, we supported and assisted his loving family in providing hospice care for Mark in their home.

After Mark's death, I considered hospital chaplaincy work – especially pediatric chaplaincy. It is ironic that during my senior year in college I had rejected a career that held some interest for me – as a pediatrician – because I did not think I could bear to see children suffer and die. Sometimes, though, the very thing we turn away from early in life is the thing that embraces us later on.

I spent the year following Mark's death in an extended internship, exploring the vocation of a professional chaplain. Following my internship, I applied and was accepted into a residency program, where along with other chaplain residents, I did intensive, supervised clinical training and peer-based learning. Following my residency in 1998, I was offered and accepted the position of staff chaplain at Regions and Gillette Children's Hospitals in St. Paul.

Preparation for a vocation in chaplaincy is an arduous process. The Joint Commission for Hospitals has set standards for spiritual care in the hospital setting. Professional chaplains are trained and board certified in medical settings to provide spiritual assessment, as well as spiritual care and support, during the crises of injury and illness, dying and death. Chaplains often consult with patients and families making major medical decisions. There is a strong ethical component to a chaplain's work. Chaplains often assist patients and families with the integration of their personal values and beliefs into the difficult medical decisions that they must make on their own or on a loved one's behalf.

Much of our work as chaplains in major medical institutions and long-term care facilities is with people of different Christian denominations and different faiths from our own. While living out of the well-spring of our own faith and religious orientation, we pledge as chaplains to be advocates for the spiritual needs of others. While our personal ability to provide spiritual care to any particular patient or family may be limited by our own faith perspective, we are committed to advocating for and aiding patients and their families in having spiritual care that is appropriate for their spiritual needs.

Spiritual traditions which are represented by significant numbers in Minneapolis/St. Paul include Hmong spiritual tradition, Native American spiritual traditions, Buddhism, Islam, Hinduism, Judaism, and of course, many forms of Christianity. I have been completely humbled by my encounters with people of different faiths who have expressed their confidence in chaplaincy to provide spiritual support during their hospital stay. The spiritual value that emerges out of many faith traditions in times of crisis is the value of our common humanity and the need for the presence of a compassionate listener – a companion – to witness our grief and distress.

I am personally indebted to an elderly Vietnamese man for allowing me into his life during the time of his wife's dying. I was called to the critical care unit on Christmas Eve day because this man was expressing some distress that the medical staff could not understand. When I came up to the unit, he was sitting in the family room. I asked if I could speak to him and asked if he would like an interpreter. He declined an interpreter and, in fact, spoke very fluent English. I asked him if he would be willing to tell me about his wife or express any concerns he had about her care and the care of his family. I explained to him my role as spiritual care provider. He shared with me that he realized the next day was an important religious holiday. He told me he did not know if he could care for his wife by himself.

As we talked more, he revealed the belief that all of the staff would go home for Christmas and that there would be no medical staff in the hospital to care for his wife. I assured him that, in fact, there would be many of us working on Christmas, including me. He said to me, "But you are a follower of Christ, aren't you?" I told him I was. I told him it seemed the right thing to do to work in the hospital as a follower of Christ on his birthday. He told me that in his opinion, Jesus was like a lotus flower, the least of all the flowers in the world, but the most beautiful. My encounter with this devout Buddhist man was perhaps the greatest gift I received that Christmas.

One does not have to dig deeply to find that most chaplains who love their work and feel a strong sense of call to chaplaincy are people who have been personally shattered by tragedy. Chaplains may be "wounded healers."[1] Many of us have spent a lifetime pondering and seeking the meaning of tragic events in our own lives. Many of us are folks who wrestle daily with God, who understand life and death through images and dreams – folks who don't fit nicely into our own religious traditions or prescriptions. Many of us have decided, along with the psalmist, to still praise God while asking the unanswerable question: **Why?**

People ask me, *"How do you do your work?"* Sometimes I don't have an answer for that – how to say that I feel peculiarly at home among the shattered, that I find comfort among the bereaved, that I like working in a place where life's tragic surprises are viewed as the norm instead of something that most of us could escape if we just lived well. I find it moving to rejoice with those who have transformed their lives in the face of a life-changing event, who live by faith and hope each and every day. I find it crucial to remember those who did not have the opportunity to transform their lives on this earth, but rather lost their lives through tragic circumstances.

Daily, chaplains face the reality that not every story has a hopeful ending and that God does not always seem fair or good, even to the faithful. Yet, we are called to hold out the hope that while not all disease or injury can be cured, many of our deepest wounds can be healed. In the words of William Bonadio, a 20-year veteran of emergency pediatric medicine, "Our work as chaplains is to simply 'keep the watch' faithfully, to be there when tragedy strikes, to bear witness to the struggle spiritually with forces that seem larger than we are."[2] The human spirit wrestles even with the forces of death, and prevails. For, in reality, God created the human spirit to be resilient, calling us out of death and into life.[3]

On February 25, 2009, I was finishing up a lecture for burn unit staff on the spiritual care of burn patients and their families. My pager went off and I reached down to turn it off. The message on the screen said, *"Family emergency. Call your brother."* Something in me knew I was about to become a family member…that I was about to cross over the border to the side of the stricken. I had the good sense to run to my office where I reached my brother. He was standing in the fields of our childhood home with our father's body. Our father was 80 years young, still caring for thousands of trees he planted over the 48 years since he and my mother purchased an acreage of old worn out cotton land in the foothills of the Appalachians. On the day my brother called me, our father had been hit in the head and killed by a tree limb that gave way unexpectedly. The limb delivered such a blow to the back of his head that he died cradled in his field, where our mother had found him when he did not come home for lunch.

Since my father's untimely death, our family lives in the solace of both friends and strangers to which Helen Keller referred when she wrote:

*We bereaved are not alone. We belong to the largest company in all the world – the company of those who have known suffering. When it seems that our sorrow is too great to be borne, let us think of the great family of the heavy-hearted into which our grief has given us entrance, and inevitably, we will feel about us their arms, their sympathy, their understanding. Believe, when you are most unhappy, that there is something for you to do in the world. So long as you can sweeten another's pain, life is not vain.* ♥

References:

[1] Henri Nouwen. *The Wounded Healer.* New York: Image Books. 1979.

[2] William Bonadio. *Julia's Mother.* New York: St. Martin's Press. 2000.

[3] Edited by Leah Dawn Buecker and Daniel S. Schipani. *Spiritual Caregiving in the Hospital: Windows to Chaplaincy Ministry.* Kitchener, Ontario: Pandora Press. 2006.

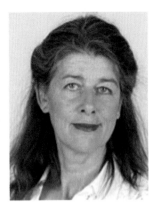

Marlou Elsen
Paulus Potterstraat 33
6523 CP Nijmegen
The Netherlands

**Phone** 031-243-600456

**E-mail** info@marlou-elsen.nl

www.marlou-elsen.nl

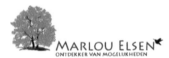

# Marlou Elsen

Marlou works as an independent organizational coach in the Netherlands, working with both individuals and teams. Her mission is to support the unleashing of the human spirit as she expands her clients' capacity to achieve their goals and dreams. Her goal is to bring real inspiration into the workplace. Marlou has an MA degree in Human Behavior. She is certified as a teacher and social worker. Marlou was also a management trainer in a telecom company and has served as a project leader for several cultural change projects. Since 1993, she has been self-employed.

# Living in My Full Power

"I lived the life that my mother lived and her mother lived.
Men made all the decisions.
We women counted for nothing.
No one ever called me by name.
I had been a daughter, a sister, a wife.
If someone came to the door and the men were away I said:
Nobody is home."

This quote by a woman in India is a huge inspiration to me on how I want to live in my full power, including being involved in meaningful work where I make a difference.

At one point in my childhood in the Netherlands, I lived at a Catholic boarding school led by nuns. My father was the mayor in my home village. As a child, outside my home and at the boarding school, I was the daughter of the mayor, not "Marlou." I was rebellious and searched for ways to follow my destiny instead of following the rules and regulations.

My mother has been an example and a model for me. When she was young, she could not attend high school; her father did not permit her to go because only boys were allowed to go to that school. She was meant to live her life as wife and mother. But that was not enough for her, so she studied at a later age. Eventually – married to my father and the mother of four children – she broke the social codes and accepted a job as a social worker.

The boarding school I attended was for girls only. The school system made me feel insecure, and I was unaware of my own potential. It took me a long time to realize I was smart! I received my diploma as a primary school teacher, but I could not see myself working at the age of 22. I had not seen anything in the world other than the small village I grew up in. I started traveling to widen my perspective. And, just like my mother, I earned a second diploma as a social worker. I chose to work with business organizations rather than with families as my mother had done.

Being a social worker in a telecom company gave me the opportunity to discover what I really wanted to do. In the late 1980s, books about the subject of coaching started arriving in Europe from the U.S. The telecom company where I worked developed coaching programs for their managers, and I was one of the trainers. Since then, I have been involved in and inspired by coaching. In 2005 I received my Master's degree in Human Behavior, and I continue to be very passionate about my coaching work!

My focus is helping clients reflect on and find their own beauty within. As they do this, they come to know who they are and begin expressing their fullest selves. This process allows them to get in touch with their internal power, and they can then move into "right action" of justice and compassion, as well as live in abundance and freedom. I am privileged to facilitate this dynamic growth process in groups and individuals.

To do this work, I must find my own inner beauty again and again. My work requires personal reflection, as well as looking at life with a beginner's mind – a fresh approach. For this reason, I like to start new projects that take me out of my comfort zone. As I put myself on the leading edge, I am able to encourage and inspire people to leave their comfort zone during coaching.

One example of living outside my comfort zone was when I lived in Nepal for several months in 2001. After trekking on my own for 28 days in the Himalayas, I stayed with a Newar family in Lalitpur (Patan), one of the three Kingtowns in Nepal. My host family included a mother and 10 children; the father and the eldest son had died. This family belonged to one of the lower castes (butchers) and they spoke Newar at home. Only the eldest son spoke some English. The children ranged from 14 to 40 years old, although they did not know their exact birth dates. Their mother was approximately 60 years old. Their Hindu religion was an important part of their life. Every morning, my host mother did *puja*, taking food, flowers, and incense to the Gods.

At one time, the grandfather of this family had owned a lot of property, but then lost much of his fortune to gambling and drinking. Now this family lived in poverty. They lived in two houses – an old family house and a small one that had recently been built. The old house had a door to the street and was built between other old houses. The ceilings were low and it was very dark inside with only small windows that had no glass in them. There were four floors; my family lived mainly on the second and third floors. Rats were part of the livestock.

The newer house, located in a courtyard, had two rooms – a small bathroom and a kitchen. I lived there with two of my host brothers. My host family owned another old house in the same courtyard that had four rooms and accommodated 15 men from India.

I met a lot of my host families' friends and relatives. I found the Nepali people to be very hospitable. Their social structure is complex – too complex for me to understand, especially regarding their forms of deference. While I was there, I experienced very different ideas about privacy – everyone entered my room to investigate everything with curiosity. In other words, my privacy was non-existent! I also experienced a big cultural difference between my idea of time and theirs. It felt like they had "no idea of time" – everything was fluid and an agreed-upon time meant nothing. They might be two hours late or they might not show up at all. They seemed to focus on whatever was in the present moment; priorities shifted constantly. The first two Nepali phrases I learned were "That is life," and "No problem." These certainly reflected their concept of time.

After two months, the situation in my host family got out of control. The eldest son started giving me orders and asking for money again and again. He was 22 years old, and in his culture he was the head of the family. Since I was now considered to be part of their family, this brother tried to exert control over me and expected me to acquiesce to him. (This was quite different from the cultural context of independence and equality I had come to know in the Netherlands.) Consequently, serious problems arose between us. I tried to communicate to get a better understanding of the situation. I saw too late how essential it is to learn the hidden codes. I hadn't been able to do this because I couldn't speak the language or even read the body language correctly. When it was apparent that our communication had completely broken down, I knew it was time for me to leave. I left my host family realizing how naïve I had been. Living outside of my "comfort zone" as I did in Nepal gave me the opportunity to learn a great deal about myself.

I believe we need to go beyond focusing on cultural differences. When we focus only on the differences that separate us, the consequence is the walls between us become thicker and thicker. I experienced this in Nepal and I encounter this in my homeland of the Netherlands. People from many different countries have relocated to the Netherlands for a variety of reasons. A lot of them are Muslims. This means we have different values and influences in the workplace and in the cities and villages where we live.

In my work in the Netherlands, I focus on altering the underlying context that shapes, limits, and defines the way each of us thinks and acts. This stretches our vision, values, and abilities. Asking questions of individuals and teams is a useful tool that can help:

- Why did we set these goals in the first place?
- What is my thinking about how I live my life and how we live together?
- Do we need to change and if so, how?

- What assumptions do we need to test?
- How can we see the situation from a different perspective?

Coaching individuals and teams and trying to affect organizational behavior can be challenging and intense. As part of my own self-care, I recently acquired a horse. His name is All frà Liberté and he is great for my work and life! From a very young age, I had dreamed of having a horse. When I turned 52, I made my childhood dream into a reality!

I am learning much about myself via riding and playing with Mr. All. He picks up on my body language, registering any incongruencies, and reacts immediately. He and the other 11 horses in the herd are teaching me to be in the present moment – focused on being calm and strong. When I am not congruent with myself or with my horse, he becomes uneasy and walks away from me or bucks. When I am calm and in balance, he relaxes. In this way, he mirrors me and provides in-the-moment feedback about my thoughts and actions.

Working with a 750-pound horse also gives me insight about my leadership ability and enhances my skills to lead. As I maintain a safe and beneficial working relationship with him and the other horses, mutual respect and trust evolve – essential skills for leadership. Furthermore, from the herd of horses I learn what it really means and feels like to be a part of a team. Working with Mr. All gives me a powerful understanding of how a misunderstood feeling, intention, or direction can make the difference between failure and success.

My horse seems to ask me again and again, "Who are you? Are you safe?" These are the same questions we ask ourselves over and over again. Asking each other these questions with awareness, respect and openness brings the right answer instead of the answer each of us *thinks* is the answer. The *real* answers provide mutually safe and beneficial working relationships; workplaces where everyone is working from their most authentic self and in their full power. That is my vision. ♥

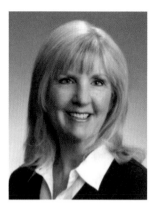

Mary Gish
Vice President/Chief Nursing
Officer
*Sierra Nevada Memorial Hospital*
155 Glasson Way
Grass Valley, CA 95945
United States

**Phone** 530-274-6165

**E-mail** mary.gish@snmh.chw.edu

www.snmh.org

# Mary Gish

Mary is a mother, a sister, a girlfriend, and has been a nurse for 29 years. She practices as a chief nurse executive in a community hospital in the Sierra Nevada foothills of Northern California, her native state. She is a complementary therapies practitioner and is currently pursuing her doctorate in nursing.

# The Green Robe

It is amazing how certain objects carry such profound meaning and emotion. As I was cleaning the hallway closet on a beautiful August day, I came across one of those special treasures. Amongst the tablecloths, empty luggage, and other items that populate this closet, was the green robe. As the floodgates of past memories erupted in my mind, I held the softness up to my face; I took a deep breath and – nothing. I was desperate for just the slightest hint of my sister, Melissa's, scent. Sitting there in the mid-afternoon light, embraced in the green robe, my thoughts turned to a similar day in August just four years prior…

Cleaning my house, I received a familiar call on the phone. "I have a medical question for you." This was how Melissa often started a phone conversation with me. In addition to sharing the trust that goes along with sisterhood, the fact that I was a nurse also reassured Melissa that I would answer most of her medical questions. I asked her what was up. She said that she had become tired and out of breath whenever she walked up a jetway; she was a proud customer service agent for Southwest Airlines. A model employee, she was full of fun and loved people! After asking a number of basic diagnostic questions, I recommended she ask for a "complete blood count" from her doctor on her upcoming physical examination later that week. She was satisfied with my suggestion.

The next Saturday I got a frantic call from Melissa's husband, Andy. He said the doctor had called them reporting on Melissa's check-up and told them that her hemoglobin was at a critical level and she needed to go immediately to the Emergency Room for fear of a possible heart attack. Without a moment's hesitation, I changed my clothes and packed a knapsack with supplies; I knew I would be spending the day in the emergency room. I had already begun the 60-mile drive to the hospital when Andy rang my cell phone and pleaded for me to come. I assured him I was already en route. So many things went through my mind as I raced to the hospital. Could it be a gastrointestinal bleed? Cancer? Your hemoglobin doesn't drop that much for just any reason. I called my cousins and sobbed over the phone, telling them how frightened I was about Melissa's situation. I let them know I needed to purge this emotion out of my system so I could be calm and strong and supportive when I got to the ER.

When I arrived at Melissa's gurney, I immediately saw the concern in her eyes. What startled me most was her skin was the color of pale white sheets and she was grey around her mouth. Dr. Smedley was the doctor on duty; Melissa nicknamed him Dr. Smelly! He recognized me from our previous working relationship and told me, "She is very, very ill." As the afternoon passed, we were informed that Dr. Kalaith, a hematologist, would be coming in to see her. (I also knew Dr. Kalaith from my past.) He briefly studied Melissa and told us that it was necessary to examine her blood cells. When he returned, he reported that her white blood cells looked very immature and that more tests were needed to determine the abnormality.

I knew what that meant – leukemia. I had hardly said the word in 25 years of nursing practice; it was a disease that was very unknown to me. In a way, I was relieved that my knowledge was minimal. I would have to follow with Melissa one step at a time on this journey. Dr. Kalaith ordered a transfusion for Melissa and the hospitalist, Dr. Mac, would admit her. Dr. Mac was one of those special doctors; you could just tell the moment you met him. He and Melissa had a very special connection. Dr. Mac stated that he would manage Melissa's care until Monday, then Dr. Blair would assume her care. I felt like we were in very good hands.

After she was admitted to a room, I left the hospital and cried the whole way home. That Sunday, I went to early morning Mass and begged Jesus to spare her. "Please make it an easy one to cure." I knew that children who have leukemia survive the disease these days. I knew that I needed to drain the fear and emotion out of my body and soul so I could be fully present on Monday when Dr. Blair gave us the diagnosis.

I was at the hospital on Monday when Dr. Blair came into the room shortly after lunch. He said to Melissa, "You have leukemia and we are waiting for further tests to determine if it is acute lymphoblastic leukemia (ALL) or acute myelogenous leukemia (AML). If it is AML you will have to stay in the hospital for 30 days of chemotherapy; if it is ALL, you can go home tomorrow and come into the office for chemotherapy." Needless to say, we were hoping for ALL. "Is it treatable?" Melissa asked. "It is curable," Dr. Blair answered. We all breathed a sigh of relief. I immediately liked him and he immediately liked Melissa. Tuesday, after Dr. Blair told us it was ALL, Melissa was discharged for outpatient treatment in Dr. Blair's office.

The following Saturday I asked my best friend, Linda, to go shopping for a wig. Melissa's chemotherapy would definitely cause her hair to fall out. Linda suffered from alopecia for several years and was a wig expert. We spent an emotional afternoon trying on wigs, scarves, and hats. I remember telling Melissa about those wonderful family members who shave their heads in solidarity for the one who would lose their hair with chemotherapy and that I would not be one of them. We all chuckled!

But I knew I would do anything I could for my sister. I had a very busy work life as a nurse executive at a community hospital and was acting as interim CEO. Even so, I made a commitment to myself at the beginning of this journey that I would spend as much time with Melissa as possible because there were no guarantees. I knew that she would always come first in my life and I would never have any regrets about spending this time with her.

The following week, she started out-patient chemotherapy in the doctor's office. I took her for her first appointment. I met all of the office staff and nurses. I was pleased to know that the registered nurse in charge was oncology certified. We brought magazines to read but Melissa was too busy answering phone calls to read them. She was checking in with everyone at work. She was the social girl. She was the last of four daughters born to my parents. She was a "change of life" baby who was born when my parents were in their early forties. She was the joy of our home, always full of fun and laughter. There may have been sibling rivalry amongst the rest of us, but we all adored Melissa. She was my baby sister, my best friend, and like a daughter to me. I was the oldest and 11½ years older than her.

After the chemo, I asked if she felt up to going to lunch. We went to Ernesto's for Mexican in downtown Sacramento, California. Afterwards we walked through a garden shop, a passion we had in common. She let me know when she became tired and I took her home. It was the last shopping trip we ever had.

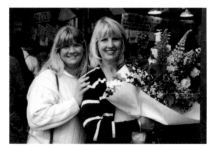

*Melissa and me*

The scheduled therapy included some heavy doses of Methotrexate. Meme, a nickname given to Melissa by my son, had to have tests to make sure that her heart would tolerate the therapy. She spent 18 days in the hospital. This was when the green robe appeared. Melissa asked Andy to purchase a "green" robe, her favorite color, and it became her hospital uniform. Over the next few months I did the best I could to support Meme in her struggles with treatment.

Later in the fall, as the Thanksgiving holiday approached, we practiced our usual routine of collecting all the November magazines and discussing new recipes for the big dinner. This year I brought the magazines to the hospital and Melissa and I talked about what we would like to try and what the family would hate. She was still hospitalized, and we were praying that her white blood cell count would reach 5,000 so she could go home for Thanksgiving. We made tentative plans by ordering the meal from the market so we could have it delivered to home or to the hospital. Finally, her lab work showed the lucky number of 5,000 white blood cells. She would be home for one of her favorite holidays! Due to her low immunity, we decided to spend Thanksgiving at her house. The whole family was present. The meal was better than home cooked that year. Some family complaining transpired towards the end of dinner. Melissa so gracefully stated in response, "Well, at least you don't have leukemia." The family members were immediately silenced. It was a sobering and insightful moment for all.

When I visited Melissa, I always tried to bring something fun to share and talk about. It was a week into December and I brought all kinds of catalogs with me. We talked about what gifts we needed to purchase, what she would get for her extended family members. It was as good as going to the mall. After this visit, she ordered all of her Christmas gifts over the telephone.

During December, Melissa was in the hospital receiving heavy doses of an experimental chemotherapy. She was very ill with high fevers. As the white blood cells decreased to zero, infections riddled her body. Andy called me one afternoon to tell me her fever was 106° F. I told him I would come down right away. The nurses were having a difficult time getting the cooling blanket to work effectively. I asked Andy, an airplane mechanic, to take a look at it. He got it working immediately. He went back to work and told him I would stay with Melissa until her fevers subsided. I started preparing ice for her underarms and groin. I took her temperature and it registered 105° F. Her nurse, Pam, came into the room. She looked rather suspiciously at me and I introduced myself. As the evening progressed, I managed Melissa's cooling blanket, ice bags, and temperature readings. Every time Pam entered the room, I gave a report on Melissa's progress. I had documented all of her temperature readings every 30 minutes for eight hours. She smiled at me and knew by the end of her shift that I was her partner in the care of my beloved sister.

It was during this time that Melissa, somewhat out of it because of her fevers, woke up crying one day. Andy and I were at her side. She said as she awoke, "I had a dream about Daddy." Our father had been gone for 15 years. She continued, "Daddy and I were sitting together on a bench and he told me that everything would be all right." I told her I thought it was wonderful to dream that Daddy had come to reassure her. Later in her journey, I reminded her of our father's words when she needed comfort.

One Sunday afternoon, I came to visit. Apparently there weren't any football games on television. (Melissa was a huge Seattle Seahawks fan!). So, Melissa had found the movie "White Christmas" with Bing Crosby on TV. I told her that is my favorite Christmas movie. She said immediately, "Mine too." I wondered how we could have been sisters for 41 years and I had not known that fact about her. I am sure it had also been a favorite of our mother's. It was a precious time – just sitting beside her, my chair next to her hospital bed, making a Christmas memory.

As Christmas drew near, it looked as if Melissa would spend it in the hospital. I knew we needed to do something special. I packed up my china, silver, and linens, and brought decorations and music. By the time we all arrived and set up the family visiting room at the hospital, it was beautiful. The table had the colors of burgundy and green drenched in candlelight. There were decorations from our homes throughout the room. The smell of cooked ham, a family favorite, permeated the air. Melissa came down from her room wearing the green robe and was amazed when she opened the door. She didn't feel well enough to sit at the table so she sat in a chair and enjoyed the quiet festivities. "For a minute I forgot where I was," she later told us with a serene smile on her face. Our Christmas celebration had been a success.

On New Year's Day, I went to the hospital to spend the day with Melissa.

I took goodies to eat and a bottle of champagne. Melissa loved wine. One of our favorite pastimes was going out to a restaurant and talking about our lives over a glass of wine. Throughout her illness, and in preparation for a stem cell transplant, she was told not to drink alcohol. She was reluctant to have even a little sip; I had to convince her that it would be all right. We shared a toast to the Year 2006.

When I arrived in her room shortly after the first of the year, Melissa didn't look well. I decided to stay with her until the evening just to keep an eye on her. Dr. Blair came into her room at dinnertime. He asked me to step outside for a private conversation. When I stepped into the hallway, he started to tell me that Melissa was not getting better and that she seemed to be succumbing to this disease. I asked him to stop telling me this information and that Andy needed to hear it from him directly. Dr. Blair told me that he thought I could communicate it better. To this day, I believe he could not bring himself to do it personally. He had gotten to know me and trusted me, but I believe he was overwhelmed with his own pain. When Andy arrived, he was not pleased that he did not hear the prognosis directly from the physician. When Andy asked me how long we would have Melissa, I told him that Dr. Blair had said it would only be a week or so. That was the most difficult day of my entire life.

I went home to pack a suitcase and made arrangements to stay at or near the hospital. Andy slept in the sleeper chair and I put my sleeping bag in a corner of the room. For the past 45 days, Melissa had been in the hospital, and during this time our relationship had deepened greatly. When I began to make calls to our extended family and friends, they began to flock to her room…my time with her was being invaded by so many. Andy stayed every night with her; I stayed off and on.

My sister never had any natural children, but she loved animals. Her favorite was Tara, her Labrador mix. In her last days, we asked the night charge nurse, Brandy, if we could bring Tara to see Melissa. With her participation in our scheme, we brought this rambunctious dog up the back stairs to Melissa's room. Melissa was so overjoyed to see her beloved pet. They hugged and chatted and said their goodbyes.

As her condition began to decline, I tried to soothe her and make her as comfortable as possible. One day I had the opportunity to bathe her. For me, cleansing her body and applying lotion to her beautiful, youthful skin was the most loving act I could do for her. I remembered when she was an infant I gave her baths, cleansed her, dressed her, and loved her. I was there to receive her when she was born and I was in attendance when God took her back home.

Before I began writing this story, I washed and hung the green robe just outside of my den. It is the symbol of my sister's brave journey of healing. Her gifts to me were her strength, perseverance, and love. Melissa touched so many lives and so many grew to love her as I do. Each day, I dedicate myself in my nursing career to her, to be better at what I do and to make a difference in someone else's life. ♥

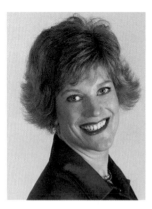

Kari Berit
*Kari Berit Presents, Inc.*
P.O. Box 2
Red Wing, MN 55066
United States

**Phone** 651-388-6789

**E-mail** kb@kariberit.com

www.kariberit.com

She is on Facebook and LinkedIn

# Kari Berit

Drawing on her background and experience as both a personal and a professional caregiver, Kari provides live and online presentations to individuals and groups interested in learning how to "start the conversations" that can successfully – and often belatedly – engage the tough issues involved in aging and caregiving. She is the author of *The Unexpected Caregiver: How Boomers Can Keep Mom & Dad Active, Safe and Independent*, as well as a popular Mental Fitness Guide (both published by the Attainment Company). She hosts a weekly radio program in Northfield and Red Wing, Minnesota, produces Caregiver Minutes for distribution online, and contributes caregiving, mental fitness, and aging articles and columns to magazines and newsletters nationwide.

She has 13 years experience as Resident Manager, Director, and Assisted Living Manager in Senior Housing facilities, and has spent over 20 years teaching and directing programs for older adults. She is also a dedicated caregiver coach.

Kari has an MS in Continuing and Vocational Education from the University of Wisconsin and a BA in Psychology and International Health Care from St. Olaf College.

# The Noble Face of Caregiving

"Why don't you come to my church and preach about caregiving," suggested my friend Jan over the phone one day. Not afraid to try something new, I accepted her invitation and headed to Manhattan, Kansas. Her pastor welcomed me and opened up the congregation to my care. My sermon title was "The Transfigured Face of Caregiving," since it was Transfiguration Sunday. I took liberty with the word and the theme, and invited the congregation to look into the face of an informal or family caregiver: that person who isn't paid to assist another, the family member who adds this new role into their already full life, or the spouse who honors their promise "in sickness and in health."

Caregiving, or the act of caring for and about someone else, changes our faces. Some of us gather deeper lines in our foreheads. Others of us lose that plumpness in our cheeks. And yet, if we can be smart about our caregiving, our faces can be transfigured, "show a *great* change, especially to something *nobler* or *more beautiful*" (Oxford American Dictionary). Being smart means we need to ask for guidance, learn about our loved one's illness, and take care of ourselves. It also means that at times, we need to set aside our emotions and simply be with our loved ones. No expectations. Just being present to the other person.

This is not always easy, especially for families. During the adult education hour at Jan's church, a discussion erupted when one woman in her 70s said, "I think our kids owe us care. Heck, we cared for them; it's their turn to care for us." Almost immediately, another 70 year old woman countered, "I don't want to be a burden. My kids have their own families now. They don't owe me anything."

After participating in the adult education hour conversation, I read in *The Star Online* (February 11, 2009) that the Chief Minister in Penang, Malaysia, believes adult children "must be accountable for their elderly parents and failure to perform such a duty will result in a failure to uphold a compassionate society. Errant children should be fined if they do not care for their aging parents." Mandating care, however, doesn't work in all families.

"What if I don't like my parents? Do I still have to care for them?" was a question I received while being interviewed on a radio show. We don't all come from happy families. In fact, many of us are products of very dysfunctional families. I could not have been a full-time caregiver to my mother. There were simply too many rules of how I was to behave that would have rendered me ineffective. But I could support her main caregiver, my father. When my grandfather needed care, I had already worked through forgiveness and was able to meet him where he was at. Now that my sister is suffering from the same debilitating disease my mother had, I've found myself caught between wanting to have her move in with me and wishing I were three states removed from her. Sometimes, there's a lot of unresolved baggage that gets in the way of giving care. When I'm able to let go of the past baggage and be in the present moment, I enjoy caring for my sister.

This isn't always the situation.

A woman who heard that radio interview later attended a seminar I was giving and when she saw me expressed a tearful, "Thank you." "My father abused me," she continued, "and I can't figure out how or if I can care for him. I am here to get clarity." She was there to get smart about caregiving, figure out if she could find a way to care for him.

But even if you have had a good relationship with your parents, the word "owe" doesn't fit with caregiving. Just as parenting our parents implies an unequal relationship, owing someone implies inequality. Caregiving is a two-way street. You give care because a parent or loved one needs help and can't function independently. What you receive back is up to you.

Not only did Jan have me preach and teach in her church, she also invited a few of her friends to her home to meet me. These friends were struggling with the day-to-day duties of giving care to a loved one. "I have little joy these days," one said to me. Jan got a phone call from one woman whose husband had Alzheimer's disease, "I don't think I can come. I've got no one to watch my husband." "Bring him along," I said to Jan.

As we were waiting for one more person to arrive, Harry, the husband with Alzheimer's disease, was sitting in a recliner. He picked up a copy of my book, *The Unexpected Caregiver*, and was reading it. (Many people assume that Alzheimer's disease robs a person of their ability to read. Not true. They may not understand or be able to recall what they've read, but most can still read, especially with a large enough font.)

The small group gathered around Jan's dining room table and I made sure I sat next to Harry. While they were sharing stories about their experiences, I spread out a deck of "Thinking Cards" (Attainment Co.) in front of Harry. (The "Thinking Cards" are part of the mental fitness tools I use in groups and one-to-ones that challenge the brain, and also assist caregivers in making connections.) Continuing the conversation, I occasionally glanced at Harry, nodding or touching his hand and looking into his eyes. Eventually, he picked up a Thinking Card. That was my cue. I paused the general conversation and tuned into Harry, "What bright colors," I said as we both looked at the picture of a hot-air balloon on the card. "Yes," he answered. I waited and he then said, "I have been on one." "Wow, what did you see?" I asked. "Everything," he answered. It's not important whether or not Harry had been on a hot-air balloon or if he even knew what it was. It's important that we connected and we could talk about whatever he wanted. The result was that Harry was included. After a few moments, and with the card still in his hand, Harry announced to his wife, "I think we should get these. They're very good."

Harry's wife was visibly tired and struggling with also raising her middle-school-aged grandson. Harry and her grandson didn't get along. When she had bought the card deck, I suggested that she spread them out as I did, and include their grandson in the "card" conversation. I also said, "It's not important that you lead them, simply let them interact over the cards."

A couple of weeks after my visit to Jan's, I received a letter from Harry's wife: "It worked. I can't believe it. They now sit around the table and try to work the cards together. I hear them laughing and am so happy and relieved that they're connecting. Thank you."

The cards in and of themselves aren't magic; rather, it's a combination of stepping outside of our emotions and tuning into something fun, non-emotional, playful. "Let go of trying to figure out why," I often tell audiences. "Simply be. Be with the person. Don't focus on right and wrong. Let go and be."

Caregiving will change us. If we are willing to learn new ways of connecting, let go of expectations and accept what is, we will be transfigured. Because we have given care, our faces will, indeed, be more beautiful. When we are fully ourselves and care from our heart, there is no more noble charge than caregiving. ♥

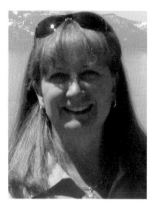

Mary Beth Schommer
208 Wellwood Ct.
Roswell, GA 30075
United States

**Phone** 678-352-8842

**E-mail** mbspirit2day@gmail.com

# Mary Beth Schommer

Mary Beth has held various positions in 26+ years in the corporate environment. She has experience in operations (domestic and international), business development, human resources, training/facilitating, and regulatory.

Healing is incorporated into her life…formally with clients, coordinating and helping at Healing Touch workshops, and by bringing healing light to every environment every day. In her spare time she loves to travel, and has visited 45 states and over 40 countries worldwide. From the heights of mountain climbing (leisurely…not the hardcore kind!) to the depths of scuba diving, enjoying what this life has to offer is her passion. She is also a minister in the Universal Life Church where she has officiated at three marriage ceremonies, thirteen renewals of vows, and one commitment ceremony.

# Thriving, Not Just Surviving,
# in Corporate America

*It all began in nineteen hundred eighty-three*
*A career in big business was all I could see.*
*What started as mundane*
*Transformed from being plain*
*When nurtured by my growth in healing artistry.*

Corporate America is slightly larger than my family; certain attributes
are common to both. Age requirements, experience, skills, etc., all play a
part in the positions we hold, whether in a business or in a family. The
nurturing characteristic of family is generally absent in big business. The
impersonal aspect of corporate life, where one is a mere number or a statistic,
can deplete one's spirit. It is often the case that, as part of a corporation, an
employee forgoes individuality in the interest of uniformity, to achieve a
smoothly operating whole. That is called surviving.

Born the youngest of nine children, with six brothers and two sisters, I
had the opportunity to participate in the "business" of a large family unit.
Many positions and duties in the family structure are determined by age
and experience. As one matures, positions change with the dynamics of
growth, as older siblings go off to college, move out, marry, join the service,
etc. As skills are learned, practiced, and honed throughout the formative

years, the repertoire of practical experience expands, preparing us for life.

When I moved from my family environment, I chose a college to attend, and then moved to full-time employment. Having graduated with a BA in Psychology helped me when working one-on-one and with small groups of special needs children over the course of the next six years. It did not, however, prepare me adequately for the rigors and bureaucratic nature of large international corporations. This was my next venture following the predominantly positive reinforcement atmosphere of the special needs arena.

After 10-plus years in survival mode at various corporate entities, I had my first "formal" exposure to energy healing in 1995. Not only was it life changing, it was life enhancing…a totally new perspective on how to live. I realized how to thrive! As my soul's thirst was being quenched, the world took on a softer tone with brilliant hues abounding.

Now what to do with all of this? I felt drawn to exploring, learning more. I was like a sponge and absorbed all the new knowledge and experiences I could. Within three years I became a Certified Healing Touch Practitioner and a Reiki Master. Book learning wasn't enough. It took me longer to assimilate the lessons and integrate this new perspective into my life – to breathe it in, believe it, and actually live it. All are essential to thriving.

Now my daily routine starts with a morning meditation which sets the highest intent for the day. I love having the healing tools with me at all times. This gives me a sense of calm throughout the most stressful day or circumstance. Trusting my healing intuition and living out of love has allowed me to cooperatively co-exist within the corporate world.

I bring energy healing covertly to work…wherever I am. Because a healing heart is incorporated into my being, it is now "in corporate!" Interactions in the workplace are now at a different level. My space in the office has become a "comfort cube" for people with headaches, stress, emotional issues, etc. When I have energetically cleared conference rooms prior to or during intense meetings, negativity has been reduced or eliminated. I have heard comments like, "She's always happy," or,

"Everything is so negative around here when you're gone."

I travel frequently for my current job (as well as for personal pleasure) and have encountered similar situations in various settings around the country. Relationships with customers nationwide are enhanced with an energetic exchange in our dealings. While it is not within corporate policy, I manage to hug my customers once we have established a relationship. Believe it or not, just as much, if not more work actually gets done from this heartfelt perspective than from a negative view of life. And it's more fun this way!

It's not easy to do this healing work in a corporate environment. Corporate life can lack energy and be very lonely at times; it's important to find a network and "plug in." Therefore, I consider myself very lucky because I am not alone at corporate. I have found a small, very powerful network of fellow healers. Even though we are all very quiet about what we do, each of us has a continual stream of people coming to our work cubicles – "just to talk." We support one another and are there for one another.

Once, when I was one of a planeload of people enduring a 7½ hour ordeal that had started out as a scheduled two hour flight, I used energy healing to diffuse stress by spreading positive energy and light around the plane. As I was deplaning, the flight attendant commented that she had never seen anything like it…everyone had remained calm and collected, with no negative interaction or confrontation. (I'm still working on flights with crying babies!)

The corporate world is focused on facts, figures, and tangibles. There is little room for the power that lies within the healing heart. There *are* sporadic glimmers of hope as individuals pursue a healing path and begin living it within corporate walls. It has been a gift for me to move from being a corporate characterless number to being the character that I am…a gift that I share with everyone I encounter. Not everyone understands there is a different way to "be." The beauty lies in watching them when they "get" it.

It is important to be true to ourselves and shine our light within the confines of not only the corporate structure but every environment we are in.

> *Living heartfelt perspective, not keeping it pent,*
> *Even within confined corporate environment.*
> *In my own unique way*
> *Throughout the course of a day*
> *Spreading my own inner light can make a big dent.* ♥

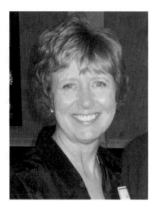

Cathi Lammert
*National Share*
402 Jackson St.
St. Charles, MO 63301
United States

**Phone** 800-821-6819

**E-mail**
clammert@nationalshare.org

www.nationalshare.org

# Cathi Lammert

Cathi is a registered nurse and is the Executive Director of the national office of *Share Pregnancy and Infant Loss Support, Inc.*

As a bereaved parent, Cathi combines her personal experience with her education and professional background as an obstetrical nurse. Her son, Christopher Michael, lived just four days and died due to Hydrops Fetalis, a complication of Rh sensitization.

Cathi and her husband, Chuck, have been involved with Share since 1983, shortly after Christopher's death. Their work began as *Share* group facilitators for the first group in St. Louis. Cathi became the executive director of *National Share* in 1992.

The part of her job that touches her most is time spent *hands on* with bereaved families and their precious babies. She feels that bereaved parents have been her greatest teachers.

# Lavender and Daisies

On August 9, 2009, my sister Margie gently left this world after a 2½ year long battle with ovarian cancer. I have experienced the death of my infant son, both of my parents, and now the death of my sister. Each loss was profound yet so very different.

When my infant son, Christopher, died I lost part of my future. When my parents died, I lost the past. But when my sister Margie died, it felt like I lost the past, present *and* future.

I am the youngest of my parents' four daughters. Margie was six years older and closest in age to me. I feel I am close to my other sisters, but Margie and I had a different kind of bond. She was more my mentor of life. Although we had some moments of discord, for the majority of our sisterhood we were close. I confided my joys, challenges, and heartaches to her. Our mother died when she was 92, and I truly thought we would both grow old like Mom and continue to share this sisterhood.

Margie's journey of fighting stage 3c ovarian cancer was not easy. She had exceptional care from the best health care facilities and doctors in the United States, including some non-traditional therapies. As a family, we watched her with awe as she courageously handled each new and often discouraging development and treatment. We all felt helpless as we so wanted to do what we could to help and support her; but she did not want to burden us and truly only wanted her beloved husband to care for her for the majority of the time.

Margie felt most comfortable with phone visits as her main means of support. She and I talked often, and I treasured those moments on the phone with her. During most visits and phone calls she really wanted to know more about me than talk about her issues, but I always tried to reverse the conversation to allow her to share about the day-to-day decisions, treatments, struggles, and disappointments. We also talked about how she worried about her dear family, and leaving them. Last but not least, she shared with me the joys in her life. Often, she was too sick to go many places, and when she did feel good she spent her days with her husband, son and daughter, and their families. I cried many tears during this time because I felt so powerless. I wanted to do more for her, yet I grew to understand her need for privacy and independence.

Five weeks prior to her death, Margie was told the cancer had metastasized to her liver and there was nothing more that could be done for her. She entered hospice home care. Her final weeks were spent in the library of her beautiful Victorian home with her *"comfortable hospice bed"* as she called it. Shortly thereafter, she realized she needed more care than her husband and children could provide, so extended family members, a few friends, and her sisters began to care for her.

It was such a gift to be next to her, to talk intimately about our past family experiences, wonder about heaven, pray together, and tend to her physical needs. It was heartbreaking some days to see her suffer. Each of us, including the hospice staff, did everything we could to keep her comfortable. She declined fairly rapidly and lived for just over a month after she began hospice care. Those final weeks I spent with Margie are moments I will cherish with all my heart for the rest of my life.

As I mentioned earlier, this loss was different from losing my son and my parents. A new journey of grief began with the death of my sister. I began to reflect on the past losses, the struggles, and how I was finally able to integrate those losses into my life. My love for my precious son and my parents has only continued to grow, and I still feel close to them. Now began the process of integrating into my life the loss I felt with Margie's death, and the anticipation of my love for her growing over time.

Several years ago after Christopher died, I began to experience his sweet presence. Those moments were profound, and often a bit overwhelming. Some people may think the events were coincidental, but it felt to me as if he was near, and this feeling aided in my healing. Sometimes, I would feel a *cheer from the stands* on a particular high or even a low day. On more than one occasion an earth-shaking event happened. Experiencing these moments of feeling my son's presence directed me to begin writing the book, *Angelic Presence*, that is a collection of short stories of hope and solace.

While there were many such experiences, one stands out as my favorite. During the first anniversary week of Christopher's birth and death, our family gathered for brunch to remember him. They lovingly blessed us with a small blue spruce. The tree was planted in our front yard, and we immediately decorated it with white lights for Christmas as it was the beginning of the holiday season. Each year we continued this tradition. We moved during the summer four years later and decided to move the *Christopher tree* as well. We asked a landscaping company to do this, and the gentleman from the company told us he would come to our house in the fall to move the tree.

On Christopher's fifth birthday that same gentleman called and said he was going to move the tree sometime soon. Four days later, on the fifth anniversary of Christopher's death, the gentleman from the landscaping company stood on my front porch with the Christopher tree. Of course, I was overwhelmed, and so was he when he learned the significance of the day. Christopher's presence was truly there with us! The Christopher tree was re-planted and we tearfully decorated it that night. We have continued to decorate the tree every holiday season since that Christmas. It now is 15 feet tall. Last year it was adorned with 3,000 lights!

I hoped and prayed that perhaps I would also feel my sister's presence in this new journey, and was grateful to experience a few such moments shortly after her death. Margie had loved both lavender and daisies for as long as I could remember. Her home had lavender soap, lotion, shampoo, all-purpose home cleaners, candles – you name it and it was lavender scented. Also, if Margie was in charge of ordering flowers when someone was sick or passed away, she always said, "Let's get white daisies."

As we were preparing for her visitation, funeral, and gathering afterwards, we knew we had to have daisies and lavender as part of her memorial and celebration. We had some challenges finding as much lavender as we needed, so I put my friends in motion. A few hours later we had several plants and cut lavender. My friends sent the most beautiful plants of lavender to the funeral home, and we decorated the reception tables with white daises and lavender as well as lavender candles. It was so beautiful, and it smelled like Margie.

As we walked up the steps toward the church the morning of the funeral, we were awe-struck by an incredibly beautiful garden of full blooming lavender. We had searched all over the city looking for lavender and here was a garden of it in Margie's churchyard! Tears flowed and we knew she was near.

A few weeks after Margie's death I had a very difficult day. I really missed her deeply. I needed to tell her the challenges of my day and I knew I could not, at least not physically. Margie was cremated, and even though I respected her decision, I was having a hard time with not having a place to go to visit her. I needed a place to visit, a place to grieve and remember her. Then I had an idea. Perhaps I could go to my familiar place of healing, *The Angel of Hope.*

Several years ago, the organization that I am the director of, Share Pregnancy and Infant Loss Support, dedicated an Angel of Hope Monument in our community for families who had experienced the death of a child. The Angel is one of 100 in the country. It rests in a sunken garden filled with budding trees, seasonal perennials, butterflies, and sweet birds. My family visits The Angel often, and Share hosts a few memorial events there each year. Each time I visit I feel comfort and peace as I remember my son while experiencing the beauty of the surrounding area. I often stroll along the walkways or just bask in the sun and pray.

Shortly after that challenging day of early grieving, we had a perfect summer day and I felt drawn to visit the Angel, hoping I could feel close to Margie there as I had always felt to my son. As I walked down the brick walkway, I almost stopped in my tracks. All around the Angel were the prettiest white daisies. Tears rolled down my face. Once again, I knew Margie was near. I stayed there for a long time, shared my heart and savored the moments.

Following my Angel visit, I went to my yoga class, as I knew I needed to renew my spirit. The class was so relaxing, and a few tears continued to flow. Our sweet yoga instructor always ends the session by massaging our necks with scented lotion as we relax. I could not believe it when I smelled a new aroma, and I smiled. Yes, it was lavender.

I will not experience growing old with my sister, but I know without a doubt she is present in the refreshing smell of lavender and in the simple beauty of a daisy…a scent and a flower and that will give me peace. ♥

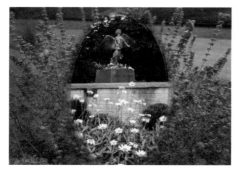

*The "Angel of Hope" encircled with*
*white daisies and lavender*

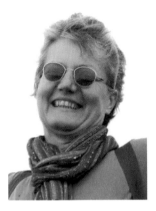

Vera Knezevic
Belgrade, Serbia

**Phone** 381-11-318-7463

**E-mail**
veraontheroad@gmail.com

# Vera Knezevic

Vera is a translator and interpreter. She speaks Serbian, English, French, and Russian, and will not get lost with her Italian and German. She has worked with humanitarian organizations and been involved with the Serbian disability movement, both as a volunteer and in a professional capacity. She is currently working for a local non-profit human rights organization called Centre Living Upright. Vera is also an amateur photographer and her work may be viewed at: http://www.flickr.com/photos/28092570@N 03/.

# From Obedient Employee to Empowered Entrepreneur

Several civil wars had torn my country of Yugoslavia into several independent states. I was 37 years old and on maternity leave with my daughter, who had severe milk-related allergic reactions as well as eczema and asthma. We had just moved to an apartment in a new suburb with cleaner air, when I learned that the federal institution I was working for had fallen apart. However, since my daughter was younger than three, my job was protected – or so I thought. The international division was the first department to be eliminated. Because I was an interpreter, I suspected I'd be next. Nevertheless, when I got my "official" notice in the mail, I was shocked. It was only days after my daughter's third birthday.

As a child, I had been taught to be obedient. My parents taught me if you do the best you can for those in higher positions, hopefully they will notice and take good care of you. Needless to say, I was an obedient employee. My employer did notice and offered me another job that would start immediately. However, because my husband worked during the day and I would be gone all day at the new job, no one would be home to take care of my daughter. With her health issues, it was not recommended that she start kindergarten before the age of four or five. To complicate things further, we had no relatives with children her age, and our friends who did have children her age lived far away. I decided to stay home with my daughter. Unemployment allowed me to spend time with her. For outings, we went to the public playground where she met other children her age.

One day, a former colleague who knew I had lost my job phoned to ask whether I would teach French to her and a friend. I had given private lessons both as a student and in between jobs, so it felt natural for me to do this. Besides, I always enjoyed giving lessons and seeing my students make progress. We began meeting once a week during the afternoon in my new students' spacious office. I brought my favorite books and newspaper articles to translate. Soon the group grew to eight people; they were emigration candidates and were highly motivated. As more asked to be tutored, lessons lasted from 5 to 8 p.m. They studied diligently and became fairly proficient…the class became a fun dialogue! For the next year, I was able to contribute financially to our household by giving the language lessons. However, as I had learned in the past, nothing is "set in stone."

With increased inflation, the combination of my husband's and my salaries wasn't sufficient to cover all of our living expenses. Furthermore, his retired aunt and uncle, who were living on a minimal pension, needed our financial support. To top it off, international sanctions were put in place and everything fueled by petroleum was either reduced or eliminated. Heating our homes became difficult, public swimming pools were closed, city buses became scarce. I worried and wondered what I could do, living in the suburbs without a car or bus transportation.

As autumn approached, some of my students left the country and the tutoring group disbanded. Every morning I took my daughter, now four years old, to a small playgroup for three hours. I decided to offer French and English lessons in the neighborhood. I advertised by putting flyers on business windows and electricity poles around our suburb. I hoped to work while my child was playing with her new friends.

Not long after I put up announcements about my services, the phone began to ring! The first call came from parents whose children needed to improve their lagging school grades. The next call came from parents who wanted their children to expand their knowledge and excel. My prices were very reasonable, and my calendar filled immediately! Although most of my students were elementary school children, I continued to work with adults wishing to emigrate. I worked my teaching schedule around caring for my daughter. For example, in the morning during her nap time I taught one or two lessons; when she was with her playgroup, I taught again. Finally, when my husband came back from work and could watch her, I would rush to give two or three more lessons.

Times were very tough; no one had much money. Clients would often pay with whatever they had – one mother offered to pay me with eggs. Even through the hardships, I regained my professional self-confidence and knew that I would never again feel scared and wait for others to take care of me. I felt empowered…this was a time in my life of saying farewell to my *obedient* employee mentality!

During the winter, I received a call from a humanitarian mission that needed an interpreter. After discussing this job with my husband and my parents, I eagerly accepted the position. It was a two-week field job that paid much better than my husband's salary. While I hadn't used my interpreting skills during my maternity leave or the two years that followed, I was excited to have the opportunity to return to work that I loved. I worked out my daughter's care – she lived with her grandparents for this short time and my husband treated her with daily lunch visits.

At the conclusion of this assignment, I was offered a different job with a mission in another city. I worked during the week and spent from Friday evening to Sunday evening with my family. This was difficult for my daughter – she missed me terribly and as I would prepare to leave, she would cling to my neck saying, "Mommy, don't go; stay with me." My heart was breaking. So, I asked my boss to give me several days of advanced vacation to spend with my family. He refused – despite my pleas. He told me that a vacation would spoil the quality of my work and it would be better for me to leave and look for a job in Belgrade. So, I resigned.

If I had been the good *obedient* employee, I would have stayed and my family life would have suffered. But now, I knew I could survive. I was willing to take risks because I knew I could provide services for those who needed and valued my expertise – and I would support my family, too. Several days later, I received a call from a Belgrade-based organization offering me a similar job.

I have lost other jobs. There is always a grieving process that happens with the ending of a position that I enjoy. But no matter how badly it hurts, it never feels as bad as that first time. I learned the most from that first devastating loss. I learned to grow from adversity and to be grateful for the new opportunities – the new doors that open – when a loss occurs. I learned to expand from being *obedient* to feeling *empowered.* ♥

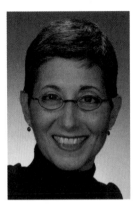

Jackie Levin
Leadership Coach, Peace
Educator & Entrepreneur
Minneapolis, MN
United States

**Phone** 612-759-7549

**E-mail** jlevin4dream@gmail.com

www.mindfulinnovation.com
includes a free e-book

www.thepowerofpossibility.com

www.butterflypeacepath.com

www.butterfly-communities.com

www.ablenetinc.com

Project M is on Facebook

# Jackie Levin

Working in business and public education settings for the past 30 years, Jackie has designed a wealth of products and programs to inspire individuals and teams to bring their full expression into "work life" and "life work."

As a co-founder of *AbleNet, Inc.* in 1985, Jackie led the development of assistive technology products and curriculum.

Jackie currently provides leadership training and development to profit and non-profit organizations through a consulting practice, *Mindful Innovation.*

In 2004, Jackie co-founded *The Butterfly Peace Path* labyrinth with sacred earth artist and corporate creativity consultant, William Grace Frost.

Jackie's community work is expressed through *Project M*, a mentoring program she founded in 2006, designed to nurture the spirit and capability of urban youth and their families.

Jackie enjoys spending time with her husband of 26 years, Rudy Rousseau, and son Michel, a college student majoring in English, Communications, and "Life."

# Project M: Daring to Dream…
# Making it Happen!

November 13, 2006

On the bus from San Francisco to Sebastopol, California, I was intently reading the assignment sheet describing the requirements for our final project. The project was part of the third of four retreats for the Coaches Training Institute (CTI) Co-Active Leadership Program.

"Look into the space of your community and your life and ask, 'What's missing? What is it that your heart cries out to contribute? What is the difference that you have been longing to make, the thing that you have been tolerating in the world?'"

My heart fluttered as I realized my tentative plan was not "right." I sighed, asking myself, "Now what?" My soul answered: "Jackie, you are here to help mentor the spirit and capability of African American boys." Time… and my body…froze as I processed once again the whisper that came from somewhere deep inside. A flash of a second later I heard another voice (the "Hater") and felt a foreboding presence that shouted: "Who do you think you are? YOU, a middle-aged, middle class white woman, have no right or ability to do this! You have absolutely no experience with urban youth. You are crazy to even imagine it!"

I felt paralyzed and breathless, yet a moment later I somehow, somewhere found the courage to stand strong and hear my truth:

"I am a visionary, a possibility thinker and a champion of the human spirit. That I know! That I can trust no matter what the circumstance!"

Deep down, I knew that healing comes when we are clear about who we are and can give our gifts freely. In that space, I connected with my calling, my soul's work, and life purpose: To be who I AM, and do what I love in the place I belong. I realized that part of my journey was to inspire others to do the same.

During that third Leadership retreat, I created a vision for my final project – **Project M**. This would be a model program of personal assets and inter-personal skill-building, incorporating a cumulative, experiential, and progressive curriculum for mentoring young African American males. **Project M** would serve youth at high risk or who had been identified as severely emotionally and/or behaviorally disordered, disengaged in school, home, or the community, and in danger of "falling through the cracks."

I saw that the foundation of **Project M** would be an opportunity for participants and mentors to answer six questions. They would share and celebrate tangible expressions of their human spirit within their home, school, and neighborhood communities by answering:

1. Who am I?
2. What do I love?
3. What am I good at?
4. What does my community love and appreciate about me?
5. What does my community need?
6. How will I help?

I knew that **Project M** would be a framework for developing positive self-identity with a holistic and nurturing approach to body, mind, and spirit. With a curriculum rich in cultural tradition that combined writing, drawing, music, movement, and drumming, every part of **Project M** would be inspired by and created for African American youth who have the wisdom, courage, and creativity to imagine their dreams and to reach their highest potential.

I am grateful for the part of me that was ready and willing to say "YES! Why not!" to this important call. I am also grateful for everyone who has come forth, ready and willing to support this journey, given that **Project M** is definitely a "takes a whole village" proposition. Most importantly, I am grateful for all of the youth who have been ready and willing to name and claim their great dreams.

Take Dante for example, a fifth grader who attended a five-day **CAMP M** during the summer of 2007.

When Dante first participated in **Project M**, he was struggling in school and was very close to being expelled. He had been labeled with a severe emotional behavioral disorder. However, it was clear that Dante was full of brilliance, compassion, and eagerness to learn. Dante's involvement with **Project M** continued into the next school year, where he participated in an exercise in which he was asked to imagine a world where he was surrounded by people who loved and cared for him. Dante drew a circle on the blackboard and wrote in the names, "Mom, Grandma, Mr. C., my principal and teacher."

The next part of the exercise involved laying a rope on the floor in a spiral shape, to represent the negative forces in life that can pull us down and get us off track. As Dante laid out the rope, he decided to label the spiral area, "the Mud." He placed a small paper heart six feet away from the spiral. Pointing out how small the heart was in comparison to the spiral, we proceeded to talk about "What grows the heart?" Dante was full of ideas… "love, family, and staying in school," among a few. For each idea Dante expressed, another "layer" was added to the heart, visually representing how the heart can continually grow, right before our eyes.

As Dante walked around "the Mud" (the spiral), he was asked to identify the negative forces in his life…"anger, peer pressure, bad choices." Yet, he recognized that we "keep on keepin' on" because we know that there is something stronger that calls us away from that area. Finally, we created a middle space called "neutral ground," a place free of pressure or expectations and where Dante could take time to think about what really mattered in his life: a place in which he could make positive choices that supported his life dreams. When the assignment was over, Dante paused thoughtfully, smiled, and said "I like it and I want to teach it to other kids." "Dante," I (Jackie) said, "You're a teacher!" He grinned from ear to ear.

Over the past three years, we've continued to develop and implement **Project M** with about 200 individuals in a variety of settings including in-school programs, after-school and summer programs, and within a series of **Project M** family evening events.

People often ask me "What does the 'M' in **Project M** stand for?" My typical reply is, "M stands for Many things...including Music, Movement, Magic Moments, the full expression of ME!, Moving beyond our comfort zones, Moms who believe everything is possible, Mentors who care and see the brilliance in our youth, Mutual support, Mystery (and the courage to follow it), and More than you could ever imagine!

I love the stories of **Project M** because they inspire me to never give up expanding the program and holding the space for hope and possibilities.

What parents have said:

"This program is the best thing that happened to me and my family."

"My kids have changed. They tell me they love me, all the time."

What the youth have said:

"I've changed from worse to good. I have stopped beating up people, stopped talking back to teachers and getting in trouble."

"**Project M** helped me with my dreams; I never knew I was a poet."

I smile when I think about two fifth-grade boys ready to sing a song at the final celebration after a three-week summer school program that included the **Project M** DreamScape Experience:

"I'm Chad and this is Kaylan. I'm going to be an inventor and Kaylan is going to be an entomologist, and if that doesn't work out, we're going to be duet singers!"

I get the chills when I remember the young boy who approached me after a simple envisioning session where we practiced imagining what we wanted:

"I have a dream," said Troy with new energy. "I'm going to contact my two sisters I've never met." The next week Troy came to me and said he had e-mailed his sisters and was going to meet them in person the next Saturday.

I get excited when I look at the photo of Shawna smiling proudly as she stands in front of her DreamScape mural, with her "I AM" words illustrated prominently down the center: *CUTE, AMAZING, SHARING, DETERMINED, AWESOME.* I think back to what I told my son hundreds of times as he was growing up: "You can be what you can see."

And, I am filled with awe when I watch the *I AM Robert Brandt* video, and hear Robert, one of the first DreamScapers, tell his story about how he took his DreamScape seriously by learning to box and committing to it. Over the course of two years, Robert's talent and dedication got him on the USA boxing team, and on his way to his dream of competing in the 2012 Olympics!

The dream of **Project M** continues to evolve from the first program for young and troubled African American boys, to current versions serving a wide range of urban youth – boys and girls – from elementary age to young adulthood. The first DreamScape was a drawing on a small poster during a two-hour session and now one version of the program is being implemented over the course of a year in six parts with a variety of DreamScape formats including murals, structures, videos, websites, journals, CDs, and more. I can't wait to see where this project will go next!

My hope is that **Project M** will continue to inspire urban youth to *imagine* a world where they can…

…experience wisdom, courage, and creativity,

…dream and hold on to those dreams, even in the face of overwhelming pressure, and,

…live a positive future where they stand strong behind their passions and talents, and bring them into our communities.

My vision is that **Project M** will continue to inspire urban youth to *know* that they are smart and to discover the secrets of life; that they can trust themselves and others who want to support them to reach their highest potential; that they can look back and feel proud of the challenges they faced and the risks they took, all for the sake of a life well lived.

As I reflect on my **Project M** journey, I recognize I AM a healer, because in doing this amazing work I get to help at-risk youth dream and plan their future. Most importantly, I AM a space-holder along with hundreds of others present and not present, who are manifesting the great dreams of our youth. Together, we hold the healing space for hope, transformation, and new possibilities. We help each other remember the power of imagining and having faith in our imagination. When we hold a vision and have faith in our imagination, anything *is* possible!

The original vision for **Project M:**
Someday every African American male in our society will be able to say...
*I know who I AM; I have a dream; I believe in ME*
*and the positive difference I will make in the world.*

...because thousands of adults in our communities were inspired to say...
*I see who you are; I share your dream; I believe in YOU*
*and the positive difference YOU will make in the world.*

... because of the African American males in their communities
who were dying to say...
*I trust who you are; I feel the dream; I believe in ME*
*and the positive difference WE will make in the world.* ♥

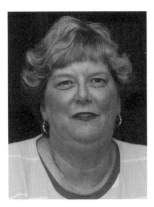

Barb Schroeder
Clinical Nurse Specialist
*Rochester Methodist Hospital*
Station 10-2
Organ Transplant Unit
201 West Center Street
Rochester, MN 55902
United States

**Phone** 507-266-7382

**E-mail**
schroeder.barbara2@mayo.edu

# Barb Schroeder

Barb has worked in various roles in nursing, including staff nurse, supervisor of an outpatient clinic, patient education coordinator, and clinical nurse specialist. For 11 years, she worked with patients and families coping with cancer. Currently, she works in the solid organ transplant field.

Barb has done program development with the *Look Good Feel Better Program*. She has been active in the community teaching *I Can Cope*, an educational program for people facing cancer. She has also been on the Board of Directors of the Gift of Life Transplant House.

Barb has given presentations locally, regionally, and nationally on the gifts of gratitude. Her goals are to bring a positive attitude to work and to look for gratitude in each day.

Barb received her AA degree from Rochester Community College and her BS degree in nursing from the College of Saint Teresa, both in Minnesota. She received her Master's degree from the University of Minnesota.

# A Journey of Gratitude

Earlier in my career, I was a clinical nurse specialist working with patients who had cancer. As part of my role, I held a weekly support group for the patients' family members. One week, a group of women were attending the support group. Although their husbands had different kinds of cancer, the women shared many of the same fears and hopes.

One woman had been in the support group for six weeks as her husband was getting chemotherapy for leukemia and he was struggling with the side effects. One day she said to the other women in the group, "I watched the best show on TV last evening. The guest on this show talked about her journey with gratitude and how it can make a difference in the dark days." I was fascinated how the mood of the group changed as the women shared how they tried to find gratitude during their husbands' journeys with cancer.

I put this idea of gratitude to rest for awhile as weeks of support groups continued. Then, on July 4th of that same year, I watched the Oprah Winfrey show, and there was the same woman talking about gratitude that we had reflected on in the support group months earlier! I said this was a *God* thing, since I commute one hour and 15 minutes to and from work each day and am very rarely at home early enough to watch Oprah. The show was life-changing for me personally, and it has influenced my nursing practice from that day on. I was intrigued by the way gratitude could help the spirit of the patients and family members I served. I had never thought about how gratitude might benefit *me*.

The next day before leaving for work, I determined I would end my day at work by reflecting on five things I was grateful for, as was discussed on the TV show. Well, the day happened, and that night before commuting home I sat at my desk. Guess what I remembered: not finding a parking place in the morning, a staff member closing the elevator door on me, an angry family member, and having too much work for one human being. I was disappointed in what had happened. *You see, if you don't look for it you will never find it.*

The next day I decided to do remedial gratitude, and the most remarkable things began to happen. I had been commuting for many years, but that morning I saw the most beautiful sunrise as I drove to work. I did get a parking place that day, and one of the staff did keep the elevator door open for me as I rounded the corner. A staff nurse said thank you to me for helping her with a difficult patient. For some reason, the day just went more smoothly! *See, if you don't look for it you will never find it.* This is true about gratitude. The difference in my two days was that, on the second day, I was purposeful in looking for the things I was grateful for.

OK, one might think, this was easy for me as I am healthy and life is good for me. How would I bring this same approach to the care of the patients and family members I served? Many were dealing with side effects from their medications, while others were dealing with life and death. I wanted to be respectful of each of their journeys, and also wanted to find a way to lighten the load. The simple thing to use is called gratitude. Webster defines gratitude as, "a feeling of thankful appreciation for favors or benefits received." "Although I may not like what is going on right now, thank you for…"

One of the patients I was seeing was Kim, a 37 year-old single mom with two children: a 17 year-old son and a 14 year-old daughter. Kim was struggling, as her treatment for leukemia required her to be in the hospital for three to four weeks at a time. She lived about four hours away from the hospital, so it was not easy for visitors to make the trip, let alone for her children to see her routinely. She missed her children. One day as we were meeting she had had it, and she began crying. I believe tears can be healing, but we also need to help find a way to see the blessing in these experiences. I sat with Kim in silence as she cried and talked about her worries and fears for herself and her children.

As we were finishing our time together, I asked her the question, "Can you share with me three to five things you are grateful for?" Kim looked at me with teary eyes and said, "I can't think of anything now." So I asked that during the next couple of days she write a list if she did think of things that she was grateful for. She was skeptical, but she said she would try. I saw Kim daily. Several days after our discussion, she said, "I have something I need to talk to you about." She had a small sheet of paper with words written on it. She said, "I thought about the discussion we had about gratitude the other day. I thought, 'What is there to be grateful for when you have leukemia, have an unknown future, and are so far away from your children and friends?'"

"At night," she continued, "when I couldn't sleep or when I was feeling alone, I asked myself, 'What am I grateful for?'" She went on, "Can I show you my list, as I did find things to be grateful for?" She brought out her list of 12 things:

- Hanging out with her children
- Dixie her dog
- Smell of coffee (couldn't drink it currently due to nausea from drugs)
- Flowers (couldn't have live flowers due to potential for infection)
- Being with friends
- Going to movies with friends
- Sleeping when it's raining
- Hearing a good song
- Watching her son play hockey

- Seeing her daughter ride her horse
- Making necklaces (which she had learned since her diagnosis and was giving them to other patients on the unit and staff)
- Making new friends while in the hospital

Some of the things on her list we take for granted everyday; but when life takes a turn, it makes us stop and reflect on little things that touch our heart and bring a smile to our face.

Patients have taught me so much about life and what is important. I thought I was helping them to find meaning in their lives by helping them identify what they were grateful for. Instead, I was the one who received the blessings of gratitude.

It has been many years since I watched the TV show with the guest speaker on gratitude. Since then, I have read every book I can find that is about gratitude. I have given many talks about finding gratitude in our daily life. Daily, I still take time to reflect on three to five things I am grateful for personally and professionally.

Yes, there are days when I still am not able to find a parking place or the elevator may close in my face, and I still work with angry families struggling with the illnesses of their loved ones. What makes a difference for me now is stopping each day to reflect on gratitude and how this has changed my day and my life.

What are you grateful for today? I hope you will take the time to stop and reflect. I can guarantee it will make a positive difference for you, and for those you love and care about. **Be Grateful!** ♥

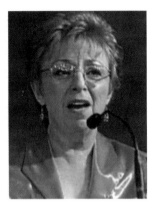

Rusty McDermott
312 North Russel St.
Mount Prospect, IL 60056
United States

Phone 847-392-6357

E-mail
Rustysangel191@gmail.com

www.onthewingofanangel.com

# Rusty McDermott

Rusty has been married to James for 41 years. They have four children and seven grandchildren. Rusty's youngest child, Meggan, was just beginning life when she was killed by a drunk driver at the tender age of 14. She remains in their hearts forever.

Music has always been an integral part of Rusty's life. While working for Advocate Health Care, Rusty had the opportunity to record a CD of music used at annual parish nurse symposiums. That music continues to be a source of strength and peace for people around the world. For 26 years, Rusty has also been a dedicated hospital minister to the sick and dying.

Rusty recently retired from her administrative assistant job at Advocate Good Shepherd Hospital in Barrington, Illinois. She and her husband love spending time and making new memories with their precious grandchildren. Rusty and Jim are avid travelers and now have the ability to travel more frequently.

Rusty is currently working on her first book about her personal transformation since her daughter died 18 years ago. She hopes it will provide support for other bereaved parents.

# A Faith Break

The world, as I knew it, ended on Sunday, November 17, 1991, at 9:44 a.m. At that moment, our youngest daughter, Meggan, was pronounced dead. At the tender age of 14, Meggan was the victim of a reckless homicide. Even now, there are no words that describe the shock and horror of that day and many to come. How could this be?

When I lost my child I lost my faith in God. My gentle husband, Jim, would later tell me, "Rusty, you had all your faith and trust in one basket, but the bottom dropped out." I would describe it as a faith break – a fracture in my foundation – a shattered heart.

I had always had a close personal relationship with Jesus…a love affair with my God, so to speak. When Meggan died, I felt abandoned, as if my God had

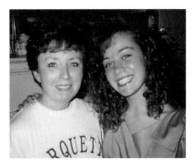

*Meggan (just months before she died) and me*

disappeared or divorced me. The question **WHY** became a pounding force within me. **WHY** did she have to lie on life support for eight days, while those who killed her lived? Her hospital room became holy ground with hundreds of people visiting, praying for a miracle. **WHY** was she not a recipient of a miracle? **WHY**, Jesus/God, did you leave us? But there was only silence. I told God, "For years I have done your will, loved unconditionally, walked with people in their darkest hours. Indeed, God, I have given of myself out of pure love. You have taken our precious daughter, but I won't allow you to take away the love in my heart. No, Lord, I will continue to love…but *not* because it is your will."

For ten years prior to Meggan's death, I was deeply committed to ministering to the sick and dying in hospital settings. I had been blessed with the gift of compassion and had always felt as if I received more than I gave.

Being present to the sick and dying is a humbling experience. Patients often told me that they felt a peaceful presence when I visited. One cancer patient looked at me one day and said, "In your eyes I see the Christ…." It was a humbling experience.

When Meggan died, I was unable to minister to anyone. Paralyzed by loss, grief, and anger, I couldn't pray, couldn't even utter "Our Father…." My rage at God drove me and became the source of my energy. On my way to mass (yes, I still attended mass!), I would scream at God, "**WHY** did you take her?" Years later, I stopped asking "**WHY?**" realizing I would never have the answer in this life. And even if I did, it would not bring Meggan back to us.

Meggan and I shared a strong bond in our love for music. I have sung in choirs and for liturgical events most of my life, and Meggan was following in my footsteps. She was gifted in piano, beginning clarinet, and had the sweet singing voice of an angel. For a long time after she died, it felt as if I had "lost" my song. Yet somehow I knew that if I was going to connect with my daughter, it would be through music. I'm not sure when the moment was that I began singing from my heart again, but when I sang, I felt "different." It was as if Meggan had left part of her gift of music with me. Often while singing now, I feel a gentle chill embrace me, and I know she is present. People tell me I have "the voice of an angel," but I know it is the blending of Meggan's angelic voice with mine – a connection between us that began in the womb.

Shortly before Meggan died, I had begun working at the Parish Nurse Resource Center. My co-workers and friends were wonderful in accepting and loving me in the darkest of my moods. One of my functions at the resource center was to assist, and often create, worship services for the annual parish nurse symposiums. In order to return to this work, I not only had to pray (and mean it!), but I also needed to sing with my heart once again.

After nine years, I was asked to record some of the music used at past symposiums. The resulting CD, *Reminiscing Through Music: The Best of the Westberg*, is a collection of the music from my heart. Today, the songs are being used at retreats, liturgical events, the bedsides of the sick and dying, for personal meditations, prison ministry, etc. Also, our precious grandchildren each have a CD and play it daily.

Creating the CD was truly a gift from God and a time of great healing for me. I feel as if this "gift" continues to bring peace, solace, and joy to others, and I am so grateful that I have been able to touch so many lives through this music. To listen to sound samples, my website is www.onthewingofanangel.com.

After several years, I returned, with great hesitation, to hospital ministry. I feel blessed not to have lost my compassion. Each patient visit brings grace-filled moments. Also, I am often privileged to assist new ministers in beginning their ministry. This further enriches my ministry.

Gradually, over 18 years, my prayer life has resurfaced, yet it is "different." I am very cautious and not always trusting. I don't believe that Meggan's death was "for a reason." Rather, I have come to believe that there is randomness to this life and that our merciful God weeps with us and puts others in our midst who provide us with His gentle presence. I know now that I never "lost" my faith, but rather, it was buried amidst the rubble of brokenness. The steps in retrieving my faith life have been painful, and often times I take five steps back and one forward. Yet, for today, I am doing the best I can with God's help and the love of my husband and those around me.

I remain reluctant to consider myself a "healer." However, others have commented how my persona reflects peace, and that I make a difference in the lives of people through my song and my presence. I believe that it is in reflecting His peaceful presence with others that the healing occurs. I am grateful to be an instrument of God. ♥

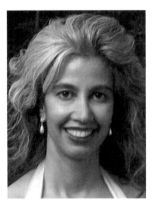

Kian Dwyer
*World Help Organization*
P.O. Box 75584
St. Paul, MN 55175
United States

**Phone** 651-353-2116

**E-mail**
kian@worldhelporganization.org

www.worldhelporganization.org

# Kian Dwyer

Kian lives in St. Paul, Minnesota. She is the owner of two businesses: *Order in the Home* and *World Help Organization*. The mission of *Order in the Home* is to create balance and space in one's home to bring peace of mind. The *World Help Organization* promotes giving freely of oneself and to others through "acts of kindness" that will change the world.

Kian hid her story for much of her life. In recent years, she has started writing and speaking out more. She is the author of *There's an Angel in All of Us* and *Living Your Chosen Eulogy: Live Today How You Want to be Remembered*, a book on how to find your true gifts and talents, and use them. She gives a percentage of the book proceeds to the Susan G. Komen Breast Cancer Foundation.

Kian holds a BA degree in Speech/ Communications with a minor in Psychology from Gustavus Adolphus College in St. Peter, Minnesota.

Her personal mission is to spread goodness and help improve the world. She encourages others to share their story, to live their chosen eulogy, release the angel within, and make a world of difference through their God-given talent.

# Daughter of Royalty

Here I sit on my haunches in the corner with my ripped up doll. All the other kids are running around wild: screaming, arguing, laughing, and simply socializing and interacting. Even though I am a warm little girl, I don't seem to do much of this with them. I intensely observe and absorb the untamed kids while caretakers meander. Instead, I am alone with my thoughts – deep, profound, mature thoughts that are way beyond my tender years. I am exercising my mind, heart, and soul, wondering how I can receive the love I desperately want and need. With perseverance, I will figure out a way to attain the tenderness, bonding and nurturing I ache for.

I think I have the answer: I will sit quietly and abide by all the rules, then they'll notice me and see that I'm the best kid ever. Unable to endure any more, I make my move. I inch toward the caretaker who is overseeing 20 children. My head is hanging down with a warm, gentle smile affixed to my face. I cling to her and begin to massage her arms and back.

My two closest friends, Susanne and Nilufar, were on the small, nostalgic merry-go-round, their favorite toy. After awhile, I would eventually join them. It seemed to be a daily event, nothing new or special.

I'll never forget the day when Nilufar shut her hand in the door. I thought she was never going to stop her screeching cry. It was actually quite frightening to see her hurt in such a way. I would frequently dream that if any kid had done wrong, then he or she would be hurt in some way or be taken away. I say this was a dream, but then again, I am not quite sure, for my recollections are hazy.

If we took our afternoon naps, we were able to go into the cool water and have an orange. I was great at faking sleep on days when I absolutely was not tired. Aah, the water felt so good on the days when the temperature would reach 120 degrees with the hot sun beating down. I guess this is the reason why all the kids had their hair cut above the ears. Yuck! I detested having to get my hair cut so short.

It is morning now, and here I am in my corner again doing some embroidery of a girl with her pet dog. I hear unfamiliar voices and look up. I see strangers, a couple, looking at me. I don't understand it...I'm scared and go back to my sewing, not saying a word. Suddenly, I am taken out of the orphanage by the couple.

Oh my! Their house was humongous. My new mother was calling for me, "Kian, would you please help with the dishes?" Misunderstanding what she had ordered me to do, I ran to the thermostat and turned it up. In just a matter of minutes, she raised her voice and pushed me against the wall. "I said the dishes, not the temperature. Will you ever learn?!" I obviously did not understand English and this family was quite impatient with me. Due to their abusive behavior, I was back in the orphanage after three short weeks.

It felt good to be back in the environment that was familiar to me. I guess broken toys and rice every day weren't too bad after all. It was a lot better than what I had just experienced. One thing I didn't like were the earthquakes we had. Everyone would scream and run under the tables. I would sit, petrified, with big eyes; my heart pounding could have probably caused an earthquake.

Two years later at age 6½, I was again sitting in my favorite corner. Oh no! There are two more strangers. Are they going to take me away, just like before? They seemed very happy and friendly, talking to the caretaker and watching all of us. My eyes kept catching their eyes...then, I'd quickly look down. I was extremely shy and didn't know how to act around strangers.

The next day, the same couple was back. I was almost happy to see them. Something about them made me feel content. They came over to me and the man asked me in Farsi (the Persian language) if I would like to go out for the day. We went shopping and out to eat.

Wow! I had never seen such a variety of toys in my whole life. Oh, what a beautiful doll! Her name was Lily and she was about 2½ feet tall with black hair and large brown eyes. Ah, look over there! There must have been over 20 different types of stuffed bears. There was one in particular that caught my eye…it was made out of lamb's wool and had a perma-smile. I couldn't believe it. I had never been so ecstatic in my entire life…they were actually buying Lily and the bear for me! How did they know? Perhaps, it was my large brown, pleading eyes.

Next, we are going out to eat. Here was my first experience with malts. I licked it first, lapping up the frostiness. Mmm, I loved it! Chocolate flavored…I just had to have another one and after that, yet another one would satisfy me even more. In the orphanage, there were set times when we ate and bathed, and they told us when to go to the bathroom. I wasn't used to making my own decisions and, consequently, after three malts I had an accident…how embarrassing! My first day out and I so wanted them to like me. I wanted them to know I wasn't bad. I found them to be caring and understanding. My "accident" didn't faze them a bit! We had a fun day. I liked my new friends. I could barely sleep due to all the excitement I was feeling inside me. I couldn't wait to see my new friends again.

It's morning again and now there is the couple watching the other kids play. Do they like them more? Finally, they come to play with me.

About a week or so had gone by and this time the same couple brought their 6½ year-old daughter named Shannon with them. Her golden hair shimmered and bounced as she came to me with a basket of candy, looked at me, and smiled. The caretaker asked me if I wanted to go with them. I responded by saying, "Mikham ba bubba beram" (meaning, I want to go with Daddy). I was wearing a cotton shift which was to be returned as soon as possible. They could have me, but not the dress.

This was my exit from the orphanage in Tehran, Iran. My new adoptive American family lived in Shiraz, Iran, which is nicknamed the garden city. They had a lovely house with a beautiful garden and seven cats. I found the cats to be such cute creatures!

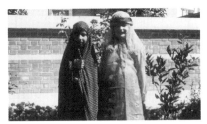
*Shannon and me on my "Adoption Day"*

Shannon had already been attending the International school in Shiraz. She had learned some Farsi through her friends, but never spoke it much until I was adopted into the family. Then she spoke it continually and we even played pat-a-cake in Farsi. She spoke it better than me; my vocabulary was terrible and I spoke only a few broken Farsi sentences. I had had no schooling in the orphanage and learned only from my peers.

Like my sister, I was now to attend school. I skipped pre-school and kindergarten and went straight into first grade. My first day, anxiously sitting in class, I clenched my aching stomach trying to hide the pain I was feeling. I stared straight ahead gritting my teeth, not telling anyone about my problem. Suddenly, the room became blurry, my head became light, and the next thing I knew, I was lying on the floor with many kids around me. I had fainted! When I came to, I wearily said I was going to get sick. My mother, who was also my teacher, grabbed the trash can.

Every day after school I went home to a tutor and sat at the table with many books. I was very interested in picture books. Showing off my English, I'd recite that the picture was a dog, a cat, or a girl. But when I was around Shannon, I would readily and cheerfully speak Farsi. Shannon didn't want to explain everything to me in English since it was difficult for me to understand and aggravating for her. Because we would be going back to America soon, my mom decided that we could no longer speak Farsi. Every time either Shannon or I spoke Farsi, we would each have to sit on a chair facing the wall at opposite ends of a large room. The first time we spoke Farsi, we would have to sit for two minutes. Each time we spoke it, the amount of time we had to sit and not say a word would increase. Finally, it came to the point where Shannon and I agonizingly sat in our chairs for 20 minutes, which is an extremely long time to sit still! We both learned our lesson and spoke only English.

On a beautiful Sunday afternoon, we were going to have a picnic in the mountains. We had peanut butter and jelly sandwiches. (My family had brought peanut butter from America because there's no such thing in Iran.) This was my first time eating peanut butter…oh, how sticky! It was on the roof of my mouth. We also had potato chips and dip. Mmm, I loved the dip so much. I carefully slid the chip into the dip, scooping up the creamy texture, trying not to break the chip. I never ate the chip because I thought it was supposed to be used as a type of spoon and not to be eaten.

As the sun was setting, our driver, Erej, drove us back in the jeep. When we returned, everyone got out and started unloading while I stayed inside. Suddenly, I was full of curiosity, turned the keys, and the jeep reversed. Everyone screamed, "Kian!" I pulled out the keys and the jeep came to a halt. This was my first driving experience!

It was now the beginning of August, and we flew to Paris to meet my new grandparents. We stayed there for six days, then rented a yellow mini bus and drove to Germany, Liechtenstein, Austria, Switzerland, and eventually into Italy and Yugoslavia. From there we flew to Greece, Turkey, and back to Iran. My grandparents stayed with us for a couple of weeks; then they went back to America, while Shannon and I went back to school in Shiraz.

I had never been outside the orphanage and I did not realize that my traveling experiences were something special. Young and very naïve, I just didn't see the importance of having the opportunity to travel around the world. I was more excited about my teddy bear than the Swiss Alps.

I seemed happy, but quiet and shy…little things impressed me a lot. I was also deeply impressed with things that affected me intimately. For example, I loved it when my grandpa joked around with me. He was trying to teach me English while we were traveling. Every time we all got on the mini bus and were ready to take off, he'd say, "And away we go!" After a while I got this into my head and said it continually.

In the middle of December, we went to Portugal and Ireland. From there we flew to Minneapolis, Minnesota, and arrived the day before Christmas. I had never experienced the festivities of the Christmas season. Everything was white and cold. I had never seen snow before; I picked some up and it slowly melted, leaving my hand cold.

After our Christmas in Minneapolis, we drove to New Jersey. This is where I would continue with first grade while Shannon would move up to second grade. School was different from that of Iran. I walked into class and everyone stared at me as I took my seat. I was the only "tan" person; what an uncomfortable feeling. At recess, all the kids would play together, but they would not include me in their fun games. I got dirty looks and they called me a "nigger" or "blacky." I was so hurt.

I was introduced to the best student in the class, Greg, who was to help me whenever I needed it. Greg was definitely a true friend, the best. He would come over to my house almost every day. On the days that I would go to his place, there would be a group of kids standing on the corner calling me names. I would ignore them, put my head down and walk briskly. They threw stones at me. Terribly frightened, I sped up my pace. After a month of putting up with this, I finally decided to tell my mother about it. She gave me directions for another way I could walk to Greg's house. It was a long way, and I was afraid to walk all that distance alone. I would often have dreams of a monster chasing me all the way home. Finally, I told Greg that he would have to meet me half-way, which worked out well.

I was also taking piano lessons and practiced every day. I didn't have many friends, but with Greg and my piano I was purely satisfied…or was I?

I was confused and deep down, I couldn't understand all that had happened in my short life. I wanted everyone to like me.

We stayed in New Jersey for only 1½ years. In 1973, we moved to Minnesota. Tears streamed down my face because I hated leaving Greg. The piano was also going to stay in New Jersey. Everything I loved was being taken away from me.

We drove to Minnesota – a very long ride – and I tried not to cry even though I was very sad. We finally arrived at our newly built house in the best neighborhood of a town called Circle Pines. The neighborhood was called "Golden Lake." One day as I was sitting in our four-level home, I heard a knock at the door. I got up and what a surprise! Standing before me was a boy who looked a lot like Greg – same color hair and eyes, and same height. I could not believe my eyes. "Hi, my name is Chad. Do you want to come out and play?" he asked. I had just come home from church wearing a dress and white gloves. Thrilled, I quickly changed into my play clothes and ran outside to play in the dirt and rocks. It was so much fun…I had a friend! Chad took me to some of his friends' houses and introduced me to Kris, Shannon, Frank, Gunner, Peter, Ray, and Eric.

Now as I lie in bed dozing off to sleep, it is 38 years later. Looking back at those years in the orphanage of strife-ridden Iran, I continue to see how fortunate I was to be one of only a handful of children ever to be adopted by Americans. I was adopted during a 1½ year test period with four American families in 1971. Since I had no family records, the Iranian government couldn't prove my religious background and I was the first ever adopted into a Christian-American family.

In fact, it was my lucky break that the Iranian government found no records of any of my relatives and that I was not born in a hospital. I was merely put in a basket at about a week old and dropped off at the police station. Later, the police put me in the Tehran orphanage, which was run by the Shah's twin sister, Ashref, and the Red Lion and Sun (similar to the International Red Cross). The Iranians were not prepared – I had no social worker and no paperwork like the other children who were adopted after me. (Suzanne and Nilufar had pages of records and the Iranian government continues to monitor their whereabouts.) I only received one piece of Persian documentation, translated into English, as my birth certificate.

Orphans, especially females, are not looked upon highly in Iran. Had I not been adopted back in 1971, I would have been married off at age 12 or on the street. (The law recently changed to nine-year-old girls being married off.) In Iran, women still walk several paces behind their husbands and men can divorce their wives and have custody of the children without their wives knowing. Women in America have more equality.

I am grateful to be in America and I often remind myself of all the freedoms we have and what we take for granted – technology, lavish cars, palatial homes, job opportunities, etc. For example, I have started two businesses and would not be able to publish the books I've written and speak as freely as I have if I had stayed in Iran.

I worked very hard at fitting into the U.S. culture and life as best as I could. My goal was to please everyone – this is what I had learned in the orphanage at an early age and it seemed to work. My inner world, however, was a stirring of emotions and I longed to find Susanne and Nilufar and re-connect with my dearest links to my early identity. Did they feel similar feelings as I did? Did they look like me? What were their memories of the orphanage? How was their life in America?

As I was growing up, I would mention to my mother that I would like to see Susanne and Nilufar. She always avoided my questions by not answering me, hoping my desire would pass eventually. Finally, in January 2000, my New Year's Resolution was to find these girls. I told my mother that I would go on Oprah's show to find them. She immediately gave me the information…she had it all along! My mother was only trying to protect me as she always had; she didn't want to give me the information in high school or college when I was more vulnerable and less mature because she knew I would have been devastated by what Susanne and Nilufar had to share.

On the same night of receiving Susanne's contact information, I was so ecstatic and nervous – I called her and we talked for four hours! I listened intently and hung on to every word as Susanne shared her memories. She had horrible memories of the orphanage. Her recollections were very troubling. (My mother had been very wise not allowing us to connect at a younger age.)

I wasn't sure if I had blocked out some memories of life in the orphanage or if I was a survivor and knew how to stay below the radar to keep out of trouble. Susanne and I shared many memories over the phone, and in person when I went to visit her in December 2006. What a reunion we had…it had been 34 years since I left her and Nilufar.

We discovered how alike we are…we are like sisters. People have asked both of us how we can be so warm and loving when we had minimal bonding and little nurturing in the orphanage. I know Susanne received her love and attention by dancing for the cooks; I received love by massaging the caretaker's arms and back. To this day, the label of being female "orphans" hasn't brought us down and it won't. We are both survivors!

For most of my life, I hid my identity and ethnic background because of fear. In 1979 (the year of the downfall of the Shah of Iran), I was threatened by my school bus driver. He was extremely prejudiced. He would drive up my driveway, swear, and say, "I know where you live." A few of the kids had reported it to school officials and, after being questioned, he was fired. Even though this incident was scary, I saw it as a good thing and it made me want to be as non-judgmental as possible. (I try to reflect this in all of my writings.)

As I got older, I longed to return and visit my homeland of Tehran, Iran. I wanted to re-experience the rhythmic music of drums, castanets, and zills, as well as eat some of the best food in the world with its unique spices of dried lime, dill, and saffron. I longed to see the caverns in the desert, the tented bazaars, street markets, and to be in the country long enough to let the culture sink back into my bones. I also felt that after a month or so, the experience would change and deepen my writing. I had a sense that I could make an even greater difference in the world.

I set up a plan to visit Iran in late September 2007. The few Persian friends I had (who still had family in Iran) were apprehensive about helping me, given the turmoil in Iran. I decided to simply Google "Queen Farah Pahlavi" and see what came up. I read through her website (www.farahpahlavi.org) and found myself immediately drawn to her healing work, especially for other women and for those who wanted to find their roots. Much to my surprise, her direct e-mail address was on her website. Could it be as simple as that to contact the Queen?! Even more unbelievable was how quickly she replied to my email…she responded immediately! She had people from all over the country calling and promising to help me find my biological family. They were wonderful, but clearly there was a misunderstanding. I wanted to see my homeland, not re-connect with my biological family. (Many years earlier, I had gotten over the fact of not knowing my biological family.)

Since September 11, 2001, there have been greater travel restrictions. I knew I needed an Iranian passport in order to be safe in the Iranian airport. According to Iranian law, once you are born in Iran you are always considered an Iranian (even if you become a U.S., Canadian, or German citizen). Once you step foot back into the country (Iran), you are considered "theirs." One of the national contacts via Empress Farah translated some information on my Persian adoption document that would make it difficult for me to enter Iran safely. I also found that the way the document was written would not allow for me to get an Iranian passport. That coupled with my being adopted put me at high risk. Adoption by Americans or foreigners has not been legal since the test period ended in 1972. The Iranian government most likely would not take the time to see that for a short period of time adoption was legal. I had many strikes against me, and Empress Farah said I should not take the risk to go to Iran.

At the time, my desire was so strong that the risk, I thought, would be worth it. I kept all this from my family, except for my adoptive father. A month later, the Empress Farah herself called me! We spoke for over an hour. Her English was perfect and she spoke so eloquently. She was beautiful inside and out. I finally asked her the question I had wanted an answer to since I was a young girl. My name, Kian (a shortened form of my full name) means "royalty." My full name, Kiandoukht, means "daughter of the royalty." I had originally thought that my name was put inside the basket by my biological parents. When I turned 18, I found out that my name was given to me in the Tehran orphanage. I had said to Empress Farah that I thought I could possibly be the illegitimate daughter of the Shah. She responded, "My dear Kian, we are all royalty. It's not the crown that we wear or the jewels that we have. It is what is in our hearts and in our minds." At the time of our phone conversation, a flood of tears streamed.

The next day it registered that she had not answered my question. She sounded so loving and warm. I truly felt as if she could have been my mother. We talked about her daughter Princess Leila who committed suicide in June 2001 at age 31. At age nine, Leila, along with her father, the Shah, and the rest of the family, was driven out of Iran and could never go back. Leila never got over the fact that she could never return to her homeland. This devastating loss is why Empress Farah continues to help people today who want to find their roots. This is the reason for her immediate response to my e-mail – my call for help.

She was honest with me and said it would be far too dangerous for me to visit Iran during its current government state. Soon after she told me this, the prominent American academic, Haleh Esfandiari, director of the Middle East Program at the Smithsonian Institution's Woodrow Wilson International Center was captured in Iran for "suspicious activities." She had been an American citizen for over 25 years and went to Iran to visit her 93 year-old mother. After several more dual-citizenship (Iranian/American) people were captured, I decided to tell my father that I would not try to visit my homeland. While he was always supportive and listened to my yearning, he was most definitely relieved that I decided not to return.

I believe that we are all here for a reason. And I have finally come to terms with why I'm here in the United States. I don't have to go back to Iran to make a difference in the world; I can do it here in America with *great* freedom and support.

My passions are speaking, writing, teaching, and being a spiritual mentor. I have been blessed to work with people ranging in age from three-year-old children to 90+ elders. As a teacher's aide at Christ Church Pre-school Learning Center in Minneapolis, Minnesota, my goal is to make a difference in 20 children's lives each year. I greet them each morning with a hug and smile, always looking forward to teaching them something new. I have always been drawn to children with special needs and I've worked with children who have autism since I was 18. From my own personal journey, I know the critical formative years are the early years. Any difference I can make in a child's life warms my heart!

By giving seminars and workshops at schools, churches, libraries, health organizations, corporate businesses, women's groups, and non-profit organizations, I hope to motivate others to take charge of their lives based on their inner values, beliefs, and moral compass. In many of these sessions, I share portions of my book, "Living Your Chosen Eulogy: Live Today How You Want to be Remembered." My intent is to model living *my* chosen eulogy, as well as offer a different perspective based on my unique cross-cultural background.

I have frequently been told my personal story is so timely for this moment in history. Once again, I remind myself that if I were in Iran, I would not have the means or be allowed the opportunity to touch and heal so many lives, by openly sharing my story and spreading kindness. I am deeply grateful and very blessed! ♥

# Voices of Vibrancy
## (the conclusion)

When my editor, Diane Maki, finished working on all of the stories, she said, "I have had this pain in my rib cage and it just went away…I just felt the healing from the women in this book!" These 31 women, from all walks of life, have shared their healing *voices of vibrancy*.

When I wrote the invitation letter to the contributing authors, I asked them to "dig deep"…to really share their hearts. This was not always easy for them; many were not used to being so vulnerable and had never seen their name or story "in print." I found myself in a role of nurturing, coaching, and encouraging. I loved working with each of them and it deepened our connection and friendship. As we moved through the process from drafting to finalizing their stories, many circled back and said, "This experience of writing was so cathartic and healing for me. I have wanted to tell my story for a very long time and I needed to find my voice. Now, I want to expand on what I started!" I can't wait to see what they individually (and possibly collectively) create next!

Mother Teresa's quote, "I have found the paradox that if I love until it hurts, then there is no hurt, only more love," is evident in these women's lives. Many have suffered great tragedies and losses, yet they continue to demonstrate resiliency and strength. Their own healing helps them to offer the gift of healing to others. They are pioneers and powerful women, deeply spiritual and spirited healers. From their stories and reflections, they model taking risks, beating the odds, being of great service, making a significant difference in the world, and living their passions. The world is a much better place because they are in it! ♥

Sending peace,

Tami Briggs
September 9, 2009

# Acknowledgements

A special thank you to:

- Each of the women who said, "Yes! I want to be a part of *voices of vibrancy.*" Your spirits are touching many people around the world.
- Diane Maki, editor extraordinaire. You "got" the passion and essence of this book from the very beginning. You are always great to work with and I value our friendship.
- Janie Delaney, graphic artist. You innately understand the bigger vision of my work and projects, then bring them to fruition with a beautiful flair.
- Michel Rousseau, intern. You have unlimited potential and are highly capable in many different areas. It will be fun to see all that you accomplish in life!

I am deeply grateful to each of you. Thank you.